New Philosophy - New Psychology - New Fitness

I'm

Core

Fit

I'm Core Fit

Success in One Day for the Rest of Your Life!

Michaelson Williams

New Philosophy—New Psychology—New Fitness

Visit our Web site at www.hwfnet.com

Printed in the United States of America

4109922

ISBN-13: 978-0615747460 (HWFnet, LLC.)

ISBN-10: 0615747469

Contents

Preface:

The information in this book comes from years of personal experience, observation of clients, and research within the fitness industry, and I draw examples from each. I use many different psychological points of view to shed light on why some people succeed and others fail in their journeys - not only to better health and fitness but to their other life goals as well. *I'm core fit* describes more than a physical attribute; it is a general philosophy that I have about health and fitness, human nature, and critical thinking. But I didn't write this book simply to give people information. I hope to provoke questions about a broken model of "service" in the health and fitness industry.

I believe generally that people do not ask as many questions as they should, particularly when they can rely on a "professional" to tell them what or how to think or which ideas and solutions to consider. For instance, we accept as a given that a doctor prescribing medication is doing so in our best interest. We trust that the mechanic working on our car is not trying to rip us off for a few extra bucks. We take for granted that a gym-assigned personal trainer is dedicated to helping us meet and exceed our fitness goals. While there may be truth to these beliefs, there is greater truth in this: You will always be your own best advocate. No one else can be as dedicated, interested, and invested in your progress as you. So this book is written to awaken an awareness that will help you understand how to be your own "professional"- in the health and fitness industry and beyond. Taking a position of self-interest doesn't mean you have to be selfish in the way you think about promoting your own wellness and longevity; but on the other hand, displaying a little more selfishness when it comes to your own and your children's health and fitness may not be such a bad idea.

The things that enhance or encourage longevity should normally be the things we protect the most, yet it seems we are protecting them less and less. We are expecting less and less. When we expect less from people who provide professional services, or from those we live with or date, work for or work with, they have no choice but to give us less. There was a time in the fitness industry when you could talk to a personal trainer who would have true knowledge and understanding of the field, and, more importantly, would have genuine interest in what you were trying to achieve. I do believe these types of people are still out there in the industry looking out for others, motivating people to do the right thing when it comes to their health and fitness. From my experience, however, I know that a large majority of the fitness industry couldn't care less about whether clients become healthy and fit. Personal trainers working within the industry – even the good ones - are often forced to put profits first, ahead of their clientele's goals and needs. When you enter a gym or fitness facility, the owners are likely not concerned about whether you're going to reach your fitness goals; they are concerned about whether they're going to be able to draft your bank account for the next 12 months. If you don't show up, all the better for them. As a paying client of a fitness facility, you must understand you do not need this type of business as much as they need you. And you should act accordingly. This is what I mean by being a little more "selfish" about your health and fitness. After all it's your money they are taking.

This attitude should extend beyond gyms and personal trainers to the rest of the "health" and "wellness" industry. Here too, from pharmaceuticals to packaged foods, we need to recognize that "the system" is designed to turn a profit, not to make you healthy or well necessarily. As a society, I believe we need to wake up and take a stand for what we know is right, but most of the time we choose to avert our eyes and pretend that there is no problem. We understand subconsciously that many of the foods we eat from the supermarkets are unhealthy for us. As a society, we are recognizing that the medicines we give to all our children have potential to cause more damage than good. We have to understand this in some manner as a collective. If we revisit our collective memory, we would recognize that years ago we didn't use so many medications and our food was free from pesticides, fertilizers, synthetic hormones, additives, and other preservatives. So much of what and how we eat and heal ourselves is based on marketing, advertising, and "product placement". Ask yourself this: What does a major food conglomerate or advertising agency know (or care) about keeping us healthy and fit in our own bodies? These are businesses, money-making enterprises that exist to make a profit off of the masses -- whether it kills us or not. Think about how odd it is that we have had to create a term, *organic*, to describe produce in its natural state! Organic is a word that never should have to be used.

With this book I hope to inspire a level of critical thinking that will assist you in seeking out information that will lead to more educated, conscious decision-making about health and fitness .Time and again I have seen clients who are heavily medicated for various diagnoses able to cut back or completely stop the medication, lose weight, and build muscle just by taking a different approach to their own health and fitness. These people who change their lives by taking an alternate path, starting a different journey through better living, eating, and exercise, create an environment within their own bodies which is no longer dependent on all of the pharmaceuticals they are prescribed. If this is the case with the few clients that I'm able to reach and re-educate, then why couldn't it be the case for the larger society? All it takes is openness to education and acceptance of a new personal responsibility for our own health and fitness.

Being *I'm core fit* has less to do with what you do and more to do with how and when you do it. It is a willingness to change, to not accept the path that you are on as fate but to change the path in order to create a new journey that leads to success and balance in life. Being *I'm core fit* is about not accepting the status quo but instead making a difference within yourself that will affect you and others in a positive manner. Being *I'm core fit* means to change your own psychological mind in order to create pleasantries instead of contradictions within your own body. We accomplish this through baby steps, minor modifications to the status quo, so small in some cases that your mind and body can barely recognize the switch from negatives to positives.

Most people assume that their health and fitness journey is going to be a difficult one. But if done properly, you shouldn't even realize that you're on a journey at all until it is complete. Weight loss, health, and fitness should be a pleasurable experience, not a chore. I believe health and fitness is all about creating balance and harmony within your mind, body, and soul in order to create a better lifestyle, which will then perpetuate positive and successful outcomes.

Author Bio

Michaelson William applies a unique philosophy and psychology when thinking about success in health and fitness. As a former Mr. North Carolina Bodybuilding Champion, Michaelson understands the physical, mental, and emotional underpinnings of success in health and fitness. He has been in the fitness industry for over twenty-five years, as a martial-arts expert, fitness consultant and author. This book distills the principles of his I'm Core Fit philosophy that he has successfully used to help clients at his local and virtual fitness studios.

Chapter 1: The Lonely Road

If you are reading this book right now you are probably on a journey to lose weight or to gain muscle. The specific paths you took to get here - and the ones you will take from here - are unique to you; after all, we each have different histories, life situations, and goals. What is the same across all of our journeys is their individuality. I call it the lonely road because the journey you are on is yours and yours alone. Most of the motivation, desire, and determination required to take one step after another along a given path has to come from within. Things and people can motivate you from the outside, but the change ultimately has to come from you. In this chapter I will detail my own personal journey, both as a means of introducing myself and to illustrate the power of internal personal drive.

My Journey

For me, the backdrop of my journey was life as the middle child and middle son of 11 children. Growing up, I drew motivation from the desire to be bigger, faster, and stronger than my older brothers. Whether it was running, throwing, jumping, kicking, wrestling or any other activity, I wanted not only to keep up, but to surpass them. But despite their constant presence and our competitions, I had to put in the effort *myself* if I was going to keep up, as I learned many times. For example, I remember clearly how my brothers and I used to race up the gravel road in front of our house. Even with a head start it was extremely difficult for me to beat the older ones. One day as we raced up the road, I could hear my brothers' footsteps quickening behind me. Digging in for every bit of strength I had, I tried to "downshift" to gather more traction and speed on the gravel. And at that moment, my hip popped out of the socket. I went down like a ton of bricks. This was neither the first nor last incident of this kind. Throughout my teens I would chronically dislocate my shoulders whenever I applied too much pressure either pushing or pulling. Many times rough-housing with my brothers would lead to my shoulder being ripped from the socket. Once my brother broke my finger; I told him he better fix it before our parents found out.

These incidents were the result of having a physical bone ailment called osteogenesis imperfecta, a hereditary condition that makes my bones softer and weaker than normal. Each dislocation event or broken bone was extremely painful, but it didn't slow me down much because I was so driven to compete with the other boys in my family. That motivation led me to study martial arts of all varieties, in an effort to strengthen the muscles around my bones – and to learn how to hold my own against my brothers. But it was another event that led me to internalize the desire to build muscle and strength that ultimately led me to bodybuilding and a career in health and fitness.

That "event" was a terrible bicycle accident when I was about 16 years old. My brothers and I were riding down the same street in front of my parents' house on our bikes. Being as competitive as we were, when we hit the blacktop road at the end of our small development, we decided to sprint as fast as our legs could carry us. I was riding a BMX bike that I had modified to make as light as it could be. My bike was the fastest, so I was able to get the early lead, even though my older brother had much greater power in his legs. I was pedaling viciously to stave off a surging attack from my brother when my pant leg got caught in the bicycle chain. There was no pulling my leg free; my foot was scraping on the ground with each pedal cycle. The only brakes I had on the bike were attached to the pedals – I had to pedal backward to apply them and this was impossible. I looked down for a split second to see how I could regain control, and then I was out. Apparently my right ankle had gone underneath the back tire of the bicycle and shattered instantly. It's a good thing our bodies go into shock because I must have been unconscious even before I hit the ground. I only remember bits and pieces after the initial accident. I was in pretty bad shape after waking up in an ambulance for a split second. When I came to again, I was in the hospital.

The injuries I sustained from this bike wreck varied in severity but stretched the entire length of my body. The skin on the left side of my face was almost completely torn off; I fractured the leaf bone which protrudes from the spinal column in the upper part of my neck; my left shoulder was dislocated (again); my left elbow was completely shattered and required two screws, one pin, and a piece of wire to reassemble. There were 24 stitches which later became 24 staples to hold the skin flaps of my left elbow back together. I had bruised ribs on one of side of my body and three broken ribs on the other side. And of course cuts, bruises, and the shattered right ankle.

This perhaps seems an unlikely entrée into the world of bodybuilding, but it turned out to be a natural progression. After my bicycle accident there were many months of rehab and hard work to rehabilitate my ankle and the rest of my injuries. I did some rehab in the hospital and follow-ups in the clinic, but the rest of the recovery was at home. Part of the rehab involved a rubber exercise band. The doctor told me to use this band to strengthen the muscles around my shoulders and arms and to use it as much as possible to strengthen everything I could. It was a plain surgical band, yellowish brown in color and fairly elastic so that I could change the resistance by shortening or lengthening my grip on the band. This simple piece of equipment helped me through my rehabilitation and was one of the first tools I used in bodybuilding and fitness. Once I saw that I could not only rehabilitate myself but build new muscle –and I could see muscles growing -- I was hooked. I wanted to get bigger, stronger and faster. My recovery from the bike accident was driven from within; I was no longer trying to keep up with my brothers, but to rebuild my body in a stronger, healthier state, for my own sake. That was over 20 years ago. Now I am a former Mr. North Carolina bodybuilding champion and a personal fitness consultant.

The moral of the story is that we can come back from just about anything. We persevere. We can motivate *ourselves* to be better, even when life deals us cards we weren't expecting. My final bodybuilding show of a ten year long amateur career was in 1999, but I have been training others since well before then. Throughout my fitness career I have trained people from all walks of life: those who were obese, professional athletes, and people with serious handicaps and disabilities. I am always looking for new and exciting ways to help my clients and others to reach their fitness goals, and that is why I have written this book.

Exploring the Lonely Road

My journey through rehab always felt like it was a lonely road. I imagine that this is what it is like for most people who have had any type of injury that requires rehabilitation – or for anyone facing a serious health challenge like obesity. Sometimes the route you're traveling is busy, but in your head you still feel alone. No one can really understand your journey. Even if a person has had similar experiences, they cannot be inside of your head or share your history and daily experiences. They can only tell you of their experiences by way of comparison. This is what I mean by the lonely road. This is your journey. Even though you may have the support of friends, doctors, nurses, or personal trainers to help you get to where you want to be, the journey to lose weight, to get fit, and to eat healthy is also a lonely road. It is a road that has to be traveled by you and for you; the journey cannot be accomplished because you want to do it for someone else. We almost always set ourselves up for failure if we want to lose weight or conquer our obesity because we want to be around for kids or grandkids or anyone else. The fact of the matter is that we need to want to be around for ourselves, not for anyone else. As much as you love these other people, it is not enough motivation to fix yourself.

Take, for example, a long-time friend of mine whose mother had throat cancer. She was a lifelong smoker, and eventually doctors had to cut a hole in her throat and installed voice box. This was devastating to her son, who is also a chain smoker. His mother made him promise to stop smoking. He vowed to cut back, to slow down, and to stop. But even seeing his mother in this state, with a hole in her throat, speaking out of an electronic voice box was not enough to get him to stop smoking. My friend's continued smoking was not because he did not love his mother or because he was not motivated by her state of being. He could not quit smoking because he was not motivated to do it for himself; he was going to try to do it because of his mother and for his mother. When he said he would quit smoking, I believed him and I think he believed himself. His heart was in the right place, but his motivation was not. Most of the motivation you have to muster up in order to succeed has to come from within; things and people can motivate you from the outside but the change has to come from you.

That's all well and good, you say, but how do you become motivated from within when you are on your own? Where do you muster the energy? How much of it is embedded into our individual psyche or disposition and how much of the ability to self-motivate is outside influence? The answers to those questions are different for different people, but I have plenty of suggestions to help you learn how to motivate yourself.

The Path of Least Resistance

For starters, let's consider that we will almost always take the path of least resistance - in our minds and bodies. No one tries to make simple chores and tasks harder for themselves or for others unless they are trying to test them in some way. We do not normally want to inflict pain on ourselves. This idea goes against our human nature. If our mind and body are always looking for the path of least resistance, we have to adapt to that and align the path of least resistance with the path we want to travel in order to accomplish our goals. What I am saying here is that the path of least resistance can – and needs to – be a path which does not lead to negative habits. When the path of least resistance is to drive through a fast food restaurant (rather than the more "difficult" path of going home to cook something healthy), where do you think that path will lead?

Many of us are oblivious to the fact we are even unhealthy because we follow this path of least resistance without conscious thought about where it's going. This "auto-pilot" behavior pushes us through many slipping points: gaining 5 pounds and then becoming accustomed to them as a natural part of our weight or our lives. People get used to carrying around the extra weight then say "It is only 5 pounds." The problem with only 5 pounds is that it becomes "only" 50 pounds, 75 pounds, 100 pounds. Obesity does not happen overnight. We do not plan for it, we don't wish for it, but it does happen. It is the destination of the path of unconscious least resistance.

This leads us to the topic of motivation. We do not really think about whether we need to be motivated to go to a gym or fitness center or even work out at home. Most of us go through our day-to-day lives without thinking about being motivated about anything, and yet there are external motivations all around us. So sitting down to watch television, though it could be unhealthy, takes no motivation at all; yet, the fast food commercial promoting "the best burgers" can motivate us to get off of the couch and do something even more unhealthy. We have so many thoughts in our heads throughout the day we do not really have time to analyze them all. If we are not analyzing all of our thoughts then some thoughts are once again on auto-pilot. If the auto-pilot is programmed for unhealthy eating or unconscious eating then how can we monitor our health and health behaviors? To start preventing the negative habits and behavior we have to start assessing our thoughts about what we are eating and whether we're exercising and being healthy. We have the ability in our minds to change the path of least resistance in order to create better outcomes for ourselves. In the chapters that follow, I will give you specific ideas for how to do this.

Chapter 2: The Road Continues

Conscious Awareness

Do we consciously make decisions about our health and fitness or are these thoughts automatic? There are times when our brains do not allow us to think about whether we're eating unhealthful foods, even if (subconsciously) we know we are. There are other times when we do consciously think about what we are doing wrong. The difference in the potential for making changes is huge. Take for example a busy mother with a hectic schedule: She drops her kids off at school by 7:30, heads to work, leaves early for school pick-up, takes one to soccer practice, drops another at gymnastics, and then picks them up and takes them home for dinner, homework, and bedtime. This schedule means she is away from the house and busy 10-12 hours a day, and in between all of this running around she has to fuel her body somehow. This woman usually makes her food choices without thinking about unhealthy eating habits; when it comes to what she puts into her mouth to fuel her body, the choice is based on convenience. In this scenario, I believe this woman does not consciously think about healthy eating, going to the gym, or anything else related to her health and fitness. Most of her thoughts are on getting her family's schedule to work each and every day of the week. This does not mean this particular scenario cannot be changed, but it indicates that this woman is unaware of the unhealthful habits she has incorporated into her schedule. She never thinks twice about eating fast food from a drive-through because her schedule is hectic, and fast food is cheap and quick. This mother puts her health and fitness behind everyone else's needs.

Now consider the same woman with the same schedule, but a few key differences. The woman in this second scenario thinks about driving through the fast food drive-through and has a fleeting thought: "This is not a good idea. There must be a different way, a different option for me." Even though she has not been on the scale in months or maybe years, she still understands her body. She recognizes that she is slowly gaining weight, her clothes are too tight, and she's had to go up in sizes. So this woman in the second scenario understands and starts to realize there's something wrong. This awareness is critical because it presents a decision-point: She can continue to go through the drive-through and pick up fast food, or she can leave the drive-through and start looking for other alternatives – an important small step towards leading a better and healthier lifestyle.

I believe that in our relations with others, there are internal sensors that tell us when we do harm to someone else and subconsciously evaluate the action as right or wrong. The same sensors can also tell us if we are doing something right or wrong to ourselves. The fundamental task we have is to recognize when these sensors are activated, understand the triggers that set them off, and do something about it. Once we recognize the triggers that motivate us to eat "bad foods", we can and must make different choices. This is our work. When our unconscious mind does not take notice to the bad habits because we have too many things going on in our life, we must try to force the conscious decisions. When we don't recognize that we are eating unhealthful foods or that we are not working out, we really can't do anything about it. But our bodies know and respond to what we eat by giving us positive or negative feedback. All we have to do is listen and pay attention to the signs in order to stay healthy and fit. Each time we get the option to behave negatively with our eating we get the same opportunity to behave positively. We have to listen to our mind and body in order to motivate ourselves into a different, positive situation.

Changing Habits

How do we change habits? More importantly how do we change bad habits? Habits are part of who we are. We get used to a certain way of doing things and they become a part of our life. In order to change negative habits we have to change our life. We have to choose and favor what is truly important over what is good for the moment. There has to be a conscious decision to make the changes necessary to better yourself. Even so, just because we make a conscious decision to change or to better ourselves does not mean we're going to succeed. So now we have to ask, "How do we <u>succeed</u> at bettering ourselves?" The answer to that question is this: **We**

have to implement small changes in our life that lead to big results. The trick is not to put the cart before the horse. A lot of people who think about weight loss think about how much weight they have to lose. So instead of thinking about how they are going to lose one, three, or five pounds, people have a tendency to focus on the fact that they have to lose 100 pounds. This way of thinking sets you up for failure right out of the gate, because when you actually start losing weight, you focus on how little weight you are losing. So if you have 100 pounds to lose and you lose two or even five pounds in the first week, the only thing you can focus on is the 95 pounds to go. This makes the journey unnecessarily long and arduous.

A key to successful weight loss is being able to manage your baby steps. If you are trying to lose a large amount of weight, train your thoughts on this: "How can I lose 5 pounds in the next two weeks?" I don't know of many people -- whether they have 5 pounds to lose or 105 pounds to lose -- who cannot accomplish losing 5 pounds in 14 days. If you are obese and you set your mind on baby steps, saying "I need to lose 5 pounds in two weeks", once you see that you've lost 8 pounds in those two weeks now you have a fresh motivation. At this point you are ready for your next baby step.

This is the mindset you should have throughout your weight loss journey until you reach your weight loss goals. Focus on one small step at a time instead of thinking about the entire picture. I don't know anyone who can open up a thousand piece puzzle and assemble it on the spot, in one sitting, just by plunking pieces on the table. But as you know, what works is dumping the pieces on the table and methodically connecting one piece to another until the form or image of the puzzle takes shape. Become your own puzzle and use the same approach. It can be helpful to use a picture of yourself when you were at your desired weight as motivation. If you do not have a picture you like, then cut out a magazine picture and place it somewhere -- or in multiple places – that you will see it each and every day. Use this picture as you would the box from the puzzle: check it often to see that you are working in the right direction, toward the desired finished product, and in order to motivate you to attain your goals.

Increasing your Motivation

Another way to increase your motivation about health and fitness is to write down the word motivation. This is another baby step to create natural positive habits for you. Once you write down the word motivation, speak to it by saying "I am motivated by _____." Write down the word motivation again and speak to the word motivation by saying, "I am motivated by_____" and then fill in the second blank. Repeat this exercise five times. Be sure to phrase your motivations as positive statements. For example, "I am motivated by not eating at a fast food restaurant this week," is a negatively-worded motivational statement about food. Replace it with something like, "I am motivated by eating something healthy every day this week." Your statement may be as simple as "I am motivated by baby steps." The idea is to slowly train your mind to do things which are healthier for you. The human mind and body can adapt to almost anything; the key is to pay attention to what you're training them to adapt to. Carry a pen or pencil with you everywhere. When you falter and you are sitting at a fast food restaurant with the food you've just ordered, I want you to take out that pen and write on a napkin, "I am motivated by my ability to throw away a portion of this meal." The key is not to have a negative attitude toward the meal, but to use it to remind you of your motivations. There is no need to add extra guilt for faltering on one of the positive motivations you wrote down previously. Just get back to the task at hand. Re-motivate yourself using the issue you are having when and where you're faltering and begin again.

Motivation and Goal Setting

When we engage in this exercise of writing down our motivations, we introduce to the mind the next step in the process, which is to use those motivations to set goals. Writing down the word motivation and completing the associated statements has laid the foundation for creating small goals upon which you can build and accomplish large goals. We often rush into goal setting, without taking the time to "prime" the mind for the what, why, and how of those goals. For this reason, I believe you should not put strict time frames on goal setting. Let the words "I am motivated by _____" resonate in your head. Let those words speak to you, create small changes in your habits, and become ingrained in your mind before you try to set goals. There is no need to rush into goal setting if you are not going to follow through to accomplish your goals. Remember, we are only looking to make small changes in order to get big results.

Minimizing Resistance

Now some may think this is moving too slowly. You should make a decision to go to the gym and to change your eating and then just do it. But I have seen this thinking in action, and I have seen it fail time and time again. Trying to build a house without planning a foundation creates more problems later. In terms of weight loss, making snap decisions and drastic changes creates more resistance to those (healthy) changes. To maximize your chances for success, we want to minimize struggle or resistance by modifying your life in ways that won't be jarring or glaringly at odds with your current bad habits. So don't even think about going to the gym. Don't think about what foods you are going to buy at the market as part of your new healthy diet. Think about what is going to motivate you just through the first change.

Think about it: most people who make a flash decision to join a gym to lose weight fail, because their decision is based on the negative motivation of having gained 5 or 35 pounds. See if this sounds familiar:

> "I need to do something about my weight. These pants are hardly fitting! I'm going to wait because the holidays are coming up and I don't want to be on a diet when everyone else is enjoying themselves."

> [Two months later.]

> "Ugh. I've gained weight from Thanksgiving, I've gained weight from Christmas, and I've gained weight from New Year's. I feel gross. I'm going to join a gym. And I'm going to make it my New Year's resolution so that I stick it out."

This is how we set ourselves up for definite failure. You have joined the gym, so you go in and get on the treadmill some week after New Year's. The gym is uncomfortably crowded because of all the other New Year's resolution new members who are trying to get on the same treadmill and work out in the same space. Crowded gyms drain your motivation because you end up not able to do what you want to do anyway. You get frustrated with the fact there are so many people in the gym and it's so damn hot. So you finally get a treadmill and you stay on there for 15 to 30 minutes. You are worn-out but you know you have to hit some weights if you want to burn more calories. You go over to the machine section of the gym and use the machines you can understand from the picture instructions, and you work out there jumping from machine to machine. Maybe if you're a little bit more knowledgeable you make a beeline for the free weights section. While over there you grunt and groan out a couple of sets here, a couple sets there, never anticipating the amount of damage you are doing to your body. You may still feel good about yourself because you have accomplished the first day and on Wednesday you are going to do it again. But the problem is, as the next morning arrives, you wake up and you cannot move because you have not worked those muscles this way since last New Year's. But you conjure up thoughts of what it was like last year when you quit the gym after a week. This year you are going to do it differently. This year you're not going to let the fitness center draft your account for an entire year before you get your butt back into the gym. These are negative motivations (using something bad to motivate you to do something good) and you are setting yourself up for failure once again. The reason? The dim light of hope.

Let's talk a little bit about the dim light of hope. Hope sounds like a positive thing, but in this case, it is another form of resistance. Imagine that hope is a light bulb that used to shine nice and bright and could illuminate the whole room. But now it's aged. This is what your New Year's resolution experience at the gym can feel like. So when you're lying in bed the day after your workout and the lactic acid has you crumpled up in the fetal position wishing you had never taken on this little task, this is another negative motivation. People have seen you in the gym; you've paid your money, so now you have to do something. Either this day or the day after you drag yourself out of bed or off the couch and you go back and you give it another shot. I would say I applaud this idea, that if you last a week or two that's perseverance, but I cannot. This "willing it through" is a dim light bulb situation. The dim light bulb always burns out. Without setting up proper motivation in taking baby steps, you become the dim light bulb that will eventually burn out. The burden of the pain, the burden of not being able to get on the equipment, the excuses you come up with to not go to the gym will all zap your energy until your light bulb burns out. You may think of canceling your gym membership, but you are likely to let it go on for months and months because you want to be there, you know you need to be there, you just are not motivated enough to be there. And at some point you get around to canceling or just let it ride until the next year.

An Example of Self-Motivation Success

They key to making that dim light bulb shine brightly is to find positive motivations that will last. What is going to motivate you to continue going to the gym? What's going to keep you motivated when it's time to eat right and correct your diet? For me, when I was getting ready to compete for the 1999 Mr. North Carolina competition, a national qualifying event on the way to becoming a professional bodybuilder, I was motivated by success. I was motivated by the fact that no one at my gym had ever won this competition. I was motivated to be that first winner of this competition. Having these motivations was essential, because it was very often a challenging road to success.

It started out okay. I had a wonderful girlfriend who kept me motivated, helped me with my meal planning, and was very supportive of me in my competitions. The problem is that dieting to a point where your body fat is three and half percent is very difficult on the mind. I remember before the competition being so stressed that I was basically unbearable to live with -- and the funny thing is I did not live with my girlfriend at the time! I was <u>always</u> hungry. I had so little body fat that I was constantly cold and had to wear long-sleeved shirts or sweaters in the summer. The feeling of being cold is due to a lack of carbohydrates to burn. The lack of carbohydrates leads to mood swings. You've heard of 'roid rage? Well let me tell you about carb rage. The lack of carbohydrates sends you into such attitude and mood swings it is like you are a different person. Because of this, we ended up ending the relationship before the competition.

Now I was truly on my own. Now I truly had to motivate myself because the road I chose was to be alone and to have no support. There were days I would sit in my apartment and just think about the end result while eating a banana, a little bit of rice, and a rice cake. I remember the agony of painting myself with an alcohol-based product called Pro Tan to darken my skin so I didn't look washed out on stage. The Pro Tan product seemed to pull the little bit of heat I had in my body right out. So I would be standing in front of the mirror trying to put on this product and I would be shivering and have goose bumps from head to toe. This went on for the next few weeks until I found myself in the hotel the night before the actual competition wondering if all of this hard work was going to pay off. I couldn't sleep, so I got up in the middle of the night and practiced poses. I had some oatmeal chocolate chip cookies and a little bit of wine to help with the vascularity in my muscles, both tricks of being a bodybuilder. Standing in front of the mirror, I felt greatness as I saw my body responding immediately to the sugar and the carbohydrates in the cookies, the vascularity changing because I was sipping on the wine.

The morning of the competition came and then it was over. I recall being backstage... being called out as Mr. North Carolina... and just hearing the crowd go wild when they called my number. The feeling of being number one, accomplishing what I set out to accomplish on the journey, and doing it on my own was the best feeling of my entire life. I won the competition that day, there was no question about it, and that night during the show people stood and applauded at my posing routines. The amount of hard work that I put into my body in order to become North Carolina State Champion paid off. And I still feel pride about not just the championship, but the journey.

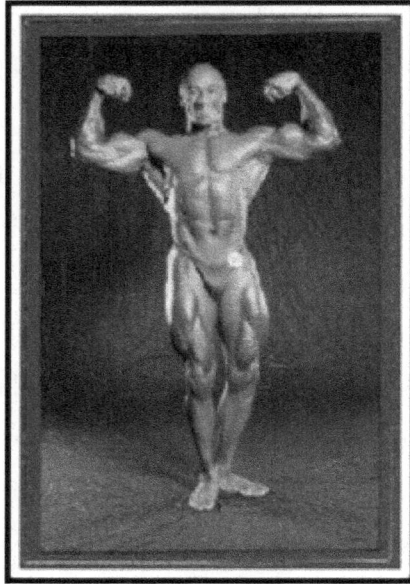

You will have your own journey. Physically, it should not be as extreme as mine, but mentally, it will be just as challenging. Your struggles will sometimes be hard. Your motivation will need to be great.

Positive versus Negative Motivation

When you are on your own journey and you are looking to win your own trophy -- whether in the form of losing 50 pounds or being able to fit into a certain pair jeans, swim a mile, or run a half marathon -- you should always use positive motivation. Positive motivation is using positive thoughts, attitudes, emotions and experiences to propel you forward on your journey. Negative motivation then, as you may have gathered by now, is using negative thoughts, attitudes, feelings or experiences to drive you. With your health and fitness, there should never be any negative motivation, only positive motivation. We can use negative motivation to get a positive result, but what fun is that? I believe that negative motivation only works in certain situations, usually if it comes from an external rather than internal source. So for example, I use negative motivation to inspire my clients to use proper form: If a client reaches down to pick up a kettle bell to do a squat and they look down at the kettle bell when beginning or ending their reps, then I make them do a punishment exercise. This use of negative motivation to get a positive result is based on my ability to watch the client and make the client get into proper form; the goal is to get them to remember the proper form. I want the discomfort of the punishment exercise to remind them to use proper form next time. Using negative motivations with yourself may not yield positive results; instead, it may result in less time working out or less time at the gym, or even possibly an injury.

Negative motivations can also sometimes turn into justifications or excuses for why you should not go to the gym or workout. Don't talk yourself into reasons why you should *not* be motivated to go to the gym or to get your workout for the day! These types of negative motivations get you negative results. You miss a day at the gym that you could have used to create a more positive outcome. There will be ordinary, uncontrollable instances that prevent you from going to the gym or making your workout, so there's no reason to add to these "misses" with excuses. Negative motivation excuses add to the number of workouts you are going to miss anyway. So use positive motivation to get you in and through as many workouts as possible and let the natural occurrences that keep you away from exercise happen without your mind interfering in the process.

Another reason to think carefully about how we motivate ourselves to get to our workouts and to eat properly is the goal setting process. As you may have experienced, once you set a goal or make a commitment to do something to better your life, it seems karma or the universe (or whatever you want to call it) puts you to the test. Setting the goal to make positive change in your life seems to come with a flip-side which is a negativity that creeps in to test your fortitude. Because of this type of karma or universal balance we should keep our minds as clear as possible of negative motivation and as full of positive motivations to help balance the scale. In our minds, if we are adding to the negative side immediately after we set a goal for ourselves, it is going to be easy to fail. Moreover, negative motivation leads to greater negativity. I believe it takes 80% more positive thoughts than negative thoughts to keep the balance at least neutral, because of the way most of us in this society were brought up. As a rule in life, try to accentuate the positive and push away the negative.

If in your life you have not experienced such a balance and imbalance, here's a test on my theory: Think about something you absolutely love - a favorite food, an object, a place, a video game or television show, anything as long as it's something that you absolutely enjoy. Now tell yourself you are not going to engage with that thing you love for one week. In less than an hour you will have a heightened awareness of that thing. So, for example, if you love vanilla ice cream and you tell yourself you are not going to eat ice cream for a whole week, I guarantee you that you'll almost start smelling and tasting the ice cream right away in your mind. On the other hand, if you can accomplish taking small steps without your brain realizing these things, you are taking away this craving and will be that much closer to your end result.

Continuing on the Lonely Road

The Role of Personal Trainers

As I discussed in Chapter 1, the lonely road is the path you have to take in order to make life changes. It may seem easier to pay a personal trainer to motivate you because then you are not responsible for motivating yourself. You are placing the burden and responsibility on someone else's shoulders. But continually giving personal trainers money to motivate you does not mean you can give up your responsibility of taking your own journey. Personal trainers are professionals, meaning that training people in health and fitness is our job, our chosen way to earn a living. We do make friends with our clients, we do spend time with clients, we do care about our clients' journeys, and we do make ourselves part of the journey, but at the end of the day it is not our journey. At the end of the day it's you who have to deal with the fact you still have horrible eating habits. It's you who will have to accept that you haven't met any of your goals. The bottom line is it's your journey alone, and personal trainers and the gym and the weights that you use are just tools to help you along your way.

Chapter 3: How do I change my diet without destroying my life?

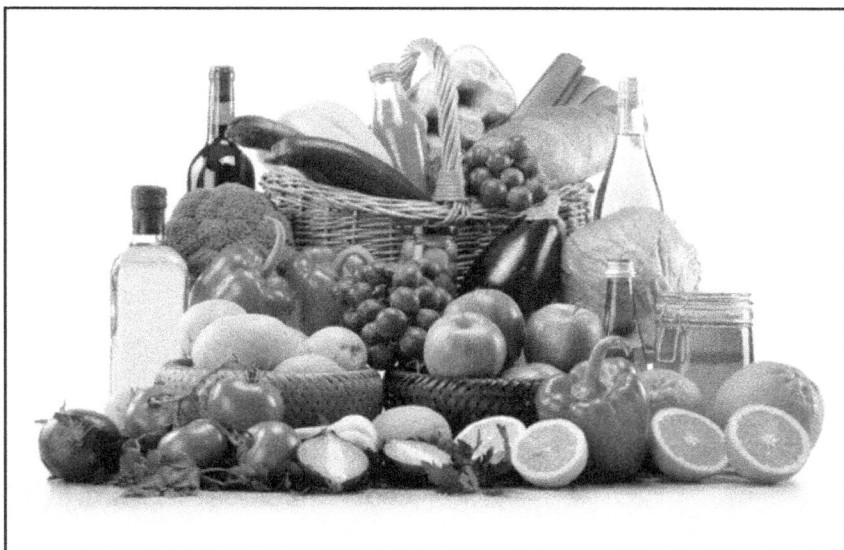

Though your journey to health and fitness is individual, you will likely have plenty of company along the way. The sad truth is this: America is fat. More than one-third of the adult population currently struggles with obesity, and that number is only increasing. To reverse the trend, nationally and individually, we have to think about how we eat and how we exercise. As we know, the equation for weight loss is astonishingly simple: calories burned must be greater than calories consumed. And yet, despite the simplicity of this equation, we continue to struggle. In this chapter, I will identify some of the main reasons for this struggle and offer tips for making this equation work in your favor.

A Simple Equation

First, let's examine the equation. We know that to burn calories, we have to move our bodies and exercise. Regular exercise of 30 or 60 minutes a day is essential to the "calories burned" side of the equation (as well as for maintaining muscle tone and bone density), but there are only so many hours in a day that we can dedicate to working out and burning calories. Given this, and the relatively greater contribution of calories consumed to weight gain, the bottom line is that you have to commit to changing your diet if you want to lose weight and change your life. If you find that statement scary or depressing, you are not alone. There is a common (though I believe misplaced) belief that diet change will destroy one's quality of life and that the satisfaction of eating and tasting food is more important than being healthy.

But there is a simple way to address this challenge and make the process easy and painless: before we change our diet, we have to change our minds. So we change our minds to change our diets to lose weight and change our lives.

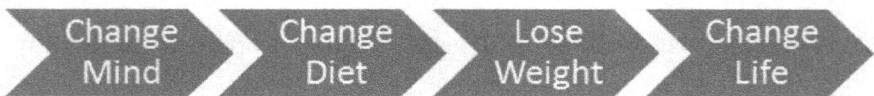

Change Mind → Change Diet → Lose Weight → Change Life

Changing your mind shouldn't seem like a daunting task. We change our minds many times each day! In this case, we change our mind to consider healthy, fresh foods as preferable and more desirable than greasy, processed, refined, and/or sugary options. We can effect a complete reversal whereby we crave the healthy option and feel repelled or disassociated from unhealthy choices. Unlike other times when we change our minds in the course of daily life, this change should be conscious and intentional, but does not need to be – and shouldn't be – an overnight process. To understand why, let's take a look at some of the mental processes and associations related to food.

Avoid "Avoiding"

None of us like to be told what to do, or that we're wrong, bad, or deficient in some way. Yet when we try to send the message to our mind that we're going to make a change to eat well, the subtext is that we're eating poorly, making poor choices, and/or doing a "bad" job of caring for ourselves. True as this may be, the ego will take offense and resist or push back against the change. You may be able to avoid your regular or favorite unhealthy foods for a week or two, but the idea that you're avoiding them makes them loom larger. So the next time you're running late or tempted to grab an old-standby snack, your ego will pop up and whisper, "Why *shouldn't* I have this [cake/cheeseburger/milkshake]? I've been so good, I deserve this. And why do I have to give this up in the first place?" The resistance, even if subconscious, creates a negative feedback loop: you feel resentment about the change, eat something unhealthy to get "revenge", feel badly about eating poorly, and then more resentment that you're being made to change in the first place (even if you yourself are the one "forcing" the change). The good news is that you can just as easily create a positive feedback loop by not forcing it and making small changes. Small, baby-step changes enable you to feel good about your small successes, which then motivate more small changes and successes. This is the idea of baby steps described in Chapter 2. By making minor adjustments to diet rather than wholesale denials or changes, you can change your subconscious mind to be aligned with your conscious/stated desire to change your diet and lose weight. Healthy eating has to slowly become normal while unhealthy eating becomes abnormal. To facilitate these changes, below I discuss four relationships we have with food, all of which have the potential to impede even small changes to mindset, diet, and weight. Understanding the relationships we have with food will help you be aware of them, so that you can use the tips provided to manage potential pitfalls.

Visual Associations with Food

There is a visual connection between what we see and how we perceive taste. We have learned to associate certain colors, shapes, and other visual cues with both flavors and judgments of taste, and, as is well known in the food packaging and marketing industries, the first taste is almost always with the eye. In several studies, researchers have removed the visual cues for taste or flavor and found that people have significantly reduced abilities to correctly name a particular flavor. For instance, when people are given gray popsicles in common flavors – cherry, grape, watermelon, etc. – and asked to name the flavor and rate its appeal, significantly fewer can name the correct flavor, and the appeal of all flavors of the popsicles declines. The purpleness of the "grape" flavor actually contributes to its "grapeness"! Again, the mind figures prominently here, storing and retrieving these associations based on visual (as well as olfactory) cues. For instance, when you see an ad on television for a juicy cheeseburger with all the fixin's, along with some perfectly crisp french fries and a cool creamy milkshake, your reaction is likely, "Mmmm!" The image of those foods is correlated with good taste in your mind. You may even feel a hunger or craving for these items simply based on reading these descriptions.

The presentation of food and perceptions of taste also go hand in hand. You are probably familiar with one of the many cooking shows on TV today. The way the chefs prepare and present their dishes on these shows is likely different than how you do so in your own home. When the featured recipe is complete and plated – even if it is composed entirely of vegetables, lean protein, or other "unglamorous" healthy foods – the careful and appealing presentation of the dish is attractive to our eyes, which signals positive associations to the mind. "This looks so good and tasty!" Perhaps its teriyaki salmon with a side of spinach and quinoa – not something that makes your mouth water when you read the words. But presented elegantly, with an herb garnish or drizzle of the marinade, this meal *looks* delicious and your taste buds are primed to experience it as such. When we recognize these visual associations, we can use them to our advantage.

The Power of Visual Associations

To get a better idea of the power of visual associations, you can do a little experiment right in your own kitchen. Mix up some cake batter according to the usual recipe. Then, add way too much salt, something like a half cup (substitute out some sugar to maintain the right consistency). Bake the cake and then frost it once it cools. Place the finished product right in front of you. When your eyes look at the finished product, this beautiful cake, you will likely be drawn to it with an urge to eat a slice -- even though you know that there was an extra half cup of salt in the batter!! The reason these urges to eat the overly salted cake do not go away is because of association. When you're sitting at the table looking at this cake, you're associating the cake with good taste.

If you want to take the experiment a little bit further, cut yourself a nice big slice of this beautifully iced cake. Try to eat a slice of cake. You'll probably throw it into the trash or spit it back out on the plate. But do not throw away the rest of the cake. Keep it on the table and try to forget about it for an hour or two. What happens when you go back in the kitchen again and see the cake? You likely will be tempted to sit down and cut yourself another slice, even though you know and have tasted how awful it is!

TRAINER'S TIP: If you want to eat more healthful foods, and enjoy them to create new positive associations, change the way you present meals to yourself. Once you make the conscious decision to change your eating habits, shop for one place setting you really like. It may be elegant, colorful, funky, or plain, so long as it is aesthetically pleasing to you. Buy one (small) plate, a bowl, a glass, and a fork, knife, and spoon. The act of "treating" yourself to something appealing alone sets up positive associations (even in the sometimes resistant subconscious mind). Then, each time you prepare a healthy meal – and only for healthy meals – present it to yourself on your new place setting as if you were a chef displaying it to an audience, complete with garnish or other flourishes if those are appealing to you. Treating your meal this way will create a positive visual that your mind will interpret as good tasting food – and eventually better tasting than the burger and fries served on foil paper out of a grease-stained bag. Again, we are not trying to eliminate fast food entirely at this point, only trying to create new, positive sensorial associations with healthy food. By focusing on presentation, we simultaneously bypass the ego's rejection of change and appeal to its pleasure centers aesthetically. This is an inexpensive way to start retraining your brain and taste buds toward a healthier style of eating. You don't have to be a gourmet chef, use fancy ingredients, or have restaurant experience – simply pick a place setting you like and use it only for healthy meals.

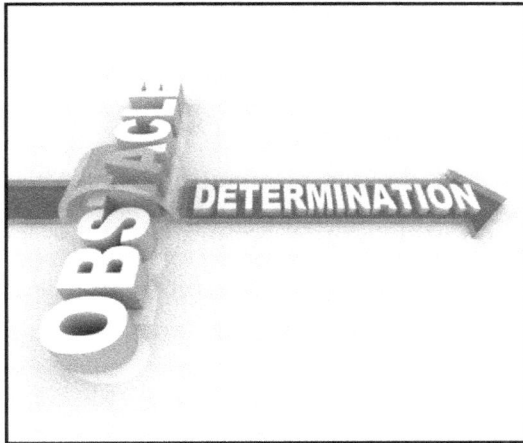

Habitual Associations with Food

Sometimes when we are not aware of our eating choices or diet, we create habitual or ritual eating patterns. It may be that every morning starts with coffee or a soda, or that you have a snack from the vending machine after lunch every day, or a bowl of ice cream after the kids are in bed each night. Whatever it is, the sign of habitual eating is the lack of decision-making about it; the decision has been made so many times in the past, at the same time/place, that the brain is on auto-pilot. "8:00pm – time for ice cream," or "We're at the mall and we always get a cinnamon roll at the mall." There is little consideration for whether you really even *want* the ice cream or cinnamon roll (or what it would feel like to skip it)– the craving has already been triggered by the habitual association of time or place and the food item.

There are two issues here with regard to changing your food planning. The first is the unconscious consumption of empty calories. With habitual association, we don't even necessarily get pleasure from what we're eating because we're putting hand to mouth in a rote or unthinking way. If you're having an afternoon snack of potato chips just because you always have that for your afternoon snack, are you enjoying them? Do you taste them? Are you even hungry? Sometimes habitual foods serve a psychological function – a break from or reward for the daily grind. In either case, consider ways to take a break or reward yourself that does not involve food.

The other issue with habitual eating is that maybe you are eating the same unhealthy food each day or in a routine because you really *do* enjoy it. Maybe Friday nights are ice cream night and you look forward to selecting your flavor as a way to celebrate the weekend. You only eat ice cream once a week and enjoy the flavors and experience when you do. As we discussed, we don't want to eliminate foods, only make small changes.

TRAINER'S TIP: For habitual eating that you do consciously enjoy, consider changing the time of day when you eat your "habitual" food.   So if Fridays are for ice cream, eat it in the morning (Friday or Saturday) instead of at night.   This may sound unusual, but it serves two purposes.   First, it disrupts the habit, making you aware of your food choices.   Secondly, eating calorie-dense foods in the morning gives your body a chance to metabolize that food energy over the course of the day, rather than having it sit all night.   The flavors and richness of ice cream are the same no matter what time you eat it, but its effects on your weight are not.

More generally, you can change the time when you eat your most unhealthy meals or snacks from after 12:00 noon to before 12:00 noon.   So if you take the worst meal or snack you eat throughout the day and move it to your first or second meal, your body will have time to metabolize or process the meal into fuel in order to be able to burn it off. This means the ice cream or cake or cheeseburger and fries can have a better chance of being burned off through your natural daily movement. The simple fact that your eyes are open and your brain is working because of interaction with other people and things put you in a better state for metabolizing unhealthy foods than if you were lying down to go to bed after a meal. If you eat the unhealthy meals at five, six, or seven o'clock at night and then sit down to watch TV before you go to bed, the effects are negative. When we go to bed, we enter a "rest state" of metabolizing our last meal. The last meal is usually the worst meal and most unhealthy meal of the day for a lot of people because it's coupled with a dessert and sometimes an after dinner snack after the dessert. Then we lay down on this food because it makes us tired and for the most part all it can do is process slowly into our fat storage centers. Don't worry - ice cream, cake or a burger and fries taste just as good at 9:00 AM as it does at 9:00 PM, so you will have the "moment on your lips" but *you'll be reducing* the "lifetime on your hips".

Food Addictions

Sometimes the habitual or ritualistic consumption of a food becomes an addiction – something we physically or psychologically *need* (or perceive we need) to get through the day. Take a client of mine who we'll call Al. Al *has* to drink Mountain Dew every single morning, and I believe he drinks up to two liters during the course of a day. In my opinion, that level of consumption is an addiction. I'm always talking to Al about the possible negative effects of drinking this unnaturally neon yellow liquid each day, but to no avail. This particular client is very fit, strong, and has low body fat. But that does not change the fact that he has an addiction to a high-calorie, low (zero) nutrient substance that may jeopardize (and certainly doesn't help) his health. You may be addicted to coffee, diet soda, chips, fries, cake... anything that you feel you physically or psychologically <u>need</u> to make it through the day, but which, in terms of nutritional needs, your body does not require. So how do we handle these addictive associations with food or drink?

TRAINER'S TIP: As with other addictions, a stepwise weaning process is required. To continue with Al's example, I instructed him not to completely stop consuming the soft drink he loves and needs so much; in my opinion, going cold turkey is not the best idea. I instructed this client to subtract one quarter of what he was drinking at every sitting. So every time he went to fill a glass with Mountain Dew, he should subtract a quarter of it. I then instructed him to wait until his mind and body got used to drinking one quarter less of the soft drink before subtracting a second one quarter of the amount. I use the same principles for clients who need 6 to 8 cups of coffee every day.

The rationale behind this system is that there is enough caffeine and/or sugar in those drinks to cause a person physical symptoms such as headaches, shaking, or dizziness if they were to stop cold turkey. So when my clients have an addiction to a food or drink, I instruct them to wean themselves off of it in a manner the body and the mind can adapt to. Essentially, the body has to go through withdrawal without the mind realizing that the particular soft drink or food is being taken away. During this time of weaning I make sure I give clients enormous amounts of positive reinforcement and positive motivation. On some occasions, I may also use a little stern verbiage or tough love as motivation, with the understanding of my clients that this is because I am involved in what they are doing. I make sure my clients understand I am a part of their journey; however, keeping everything in perspective, I cannot go to my clients' homes and subtract the amount of soft drink or coffee they are drinking each and every day. I cannot do the weaning process for them. They have to take responsibility for curbing their own food addictions. I can only encourage them and motivate them.

Social Eating

For as long as humans have lived in groups, food has held a central role in the social and cultural interactions among us. Imagine any social gathering and food features prominently: birthdays (cake and ice cream); weddings (dinner, drinks, cake); cocktail parties (hors d'oeuvres and alcohol); Super Bowl parties (beer, nachos, wings, pizza); holiday parties (eggnog, cookies) and so on. I'm sure you could think of many more occasions and list your favorite foods associated with each. There is also the *"mangia, mangia, mangia"* mentality of many hostesses when you are traveling or visiting, insisting that you eat this, try this, have more of this - and then dessert! In these situations it can be socially awkward or downright rude to refuse. Changing your eating habits does not mean excluding yourself from social life. These events are important for our social and emotional well-being, and are the "highlights" of life, breaking from the normal routine.

TRAINER'S TIP: When you know one of these occasions is coming up, try to make the social event a part of your plan for the week. It's okay to have a "day off" from clean eating (see Chapter 4 for more on the ketosis day), but that day should be just that though – one day and then right back to the food plan. Manage your food plan during the week so that you can enjoy your social activities on the weekend or whatever day you choose. And remember to listen to your body. Whether you are dieting, food planning, or enjoying your "day off", make sure that you are listening to your body's feedback. It may be that it wants a lot less of those fried, sweet, or heavily salted foods than your eyes (or hostess) would tell you.

Putting It All Together

By using little tricks and tips such as creating a different table place setting for yourself or switching the timing of your favorite indulgence, you are gaining control of your eating habits and your diet. You should always think of new and creative ways to be in control of your diet and eating plans and not have what you eat (or don't eat) control you. You can lose weight without dieting. I will repeat this and you should say it to yourself, "You can lose weight without dieting." I did not say you can reach your target weight without dieting, but you can get started by making small changes, that will yield positive-motivation building results. Your diet – and your relationship to it, positive or negative - will have a great impact on how you lose weight, if your weight loss is healthy, and whether you can maintain it. As discussed, individuals who go from eating burgers and fries to eating soy and salmon may start to build resentment toward "healthy eating". Healthy eating then becomes a negative motivation and you return back to the place you started. So take small steps, as described. You now have concrete tips on the types of changes to make, a recognition of some common eating triggers, and ideas to defuse diet-downers, so in the next chapter I'll talk a little more about helping the changes that you make stick.

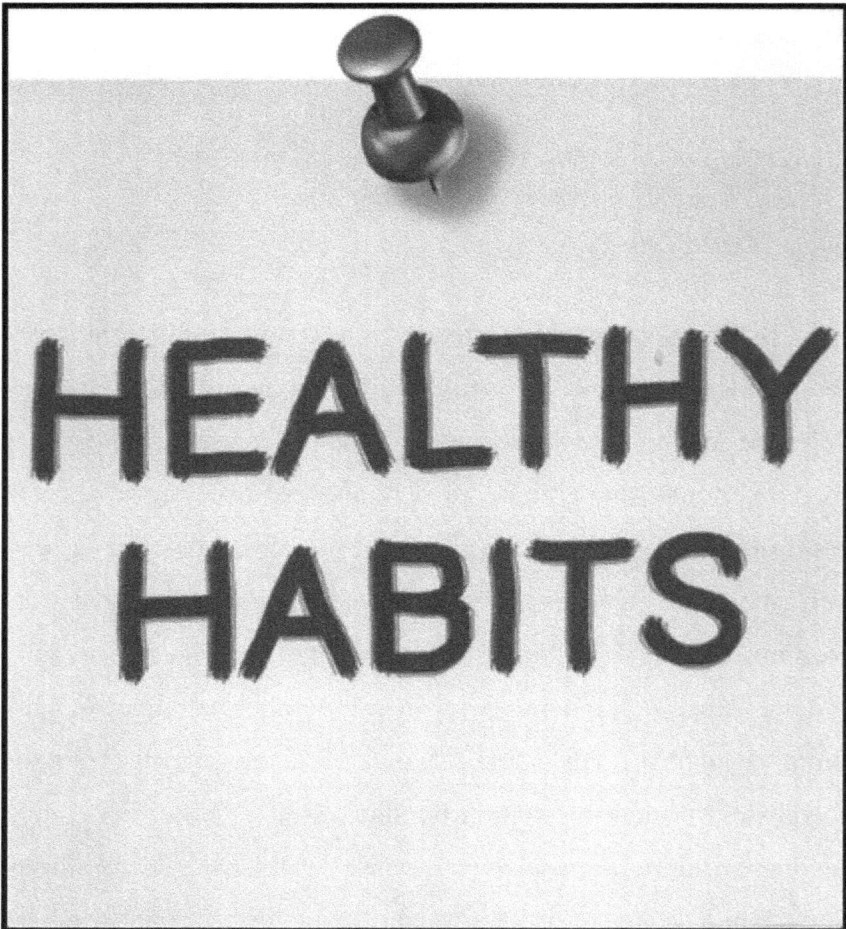

Chapter 4: Are The Habits Starting to Stick?

At some stage in the process of changing your diet, "eating healthy" has to become an afterthought. If you are overweight or obese and you have poor eating habits now, it's probably because your unhealthy eating habits are simply an afterthought. The way you eat now is not in the forefront of your mind because it's part of the habit or ritual; the conscious mind is not engaged in making decisions about the unhealthy foods you are eating. **This is where you want to get with healthy eating.** But if you were to switch and start eating healthful foods, it would then be in the forefront of your mind every single moment of that healthy meal. Eating healthy would be a conscious thought and conscious decision at every turn. You would be counting calories, measuring things out, wondering whether to eat spinach or carrots, concerned about monitoring carbohydrate intake. You would also be thinking about anything you are doing or eating that may be a setback. Any cheat or unhealthy eating you did then come to the forefront of your thinking. This type of attention to detail is also not productive. We're trying to get to the point of "auto-pilot" healthy.

Forming New, Healthy Habits

One of the ways that I inspire my clients to make changes in their lives is to institute short-term challenges that shake up the normal routine. For example, I had some of my clients follow a juicing regimen. For the first week, they juiced organic fruits and vegetables every day six to 10 times a day, to break from their unhealthy auto-pilot and create a new behavior. The premise of creating this juicing habit is that once the challenge is over, even though they're not juicing six or more times a day, the process of juicing stays in their daily or weekly regimen. If they are juicing once or twice a day, three or four times a week, then they are better off than they were before the challenge started. Notice that we have not set an unrealistic goal for clients to juice several times a day for the rest of their life because it doesn't fit within their normal lifestyle. Any changes to behavior or goals that you set need to fit into your normal everyday lifestyle or you will not treat that change as something that should be taken seriously. Not every one of my clients continued to juice after the fitness challenge was over, but that just means some people might respond better to a different type of motivation. I am constantly seeking to challenge and change the minds and habits of my clients with different methods. When you are trying to self-motivate to reach a fitness goal, you have to figure out what methods of motivation and good habit-forming behavior will work and stick for you. Don't be discouraged if the first thing you try doesn't work out; acknowledge that you have learned something about what doesn't work well for you, and try something else!

Effective Goal Setting

Above, I mentioned the unrealistic goal of juicing six or more times a day for the rest of your life. It may be self-evident that unrealistic goals are ineffective, because with them we set ourselves up for failure. If our work or school or social schedule does not permit us to be at home to juice fresh fruits and vegetables several times a day, we cannot expect to be able to juice so many times a day! We might make it one week or two, but this is not sustainable for the long term. And sustainability and timing of goals matters. For instance, if we were to set a goal for saving a certain amount of money by the time we retire; we would understand this is a long-term life goal. Notice I did not say we are saving money until the time we are 65. Those two ways of goal setting are completely different in the way your brain responds to them. When you incorporate an age or any kind of time limit on goal setting, it gives you a way out. If you are 30 years old and start a savings account for when you're 65, at 40 you could decide to make a big-ticket purchase and use that money, and start over with the saving. You could do the same at 50 or 55. On the other hand, if you set a monetary goal based on when you retire, which has no bearing on age, you don't have the out. In this scenario, if you are 30 years old and you start this retirement fund, you may have enough money to retire by the time you are 50. Goal setting this way does not allow you the out of an event or time limit. We have to understand how to frame and set our goals so that our minds focus on how the goal is supposed to be accomplished, instead of goals that stimulate the mind to figure out ways to avoid or skirt the goal.

If we stick with the same retirement savings example and drill down a little bit deeper into how the mind perceives the way you set goals, we can look at it in small chunks. If you set up a savings account and you make a deduction each week from your checking account of let's say $25, you would miss the $25 every week for a certain amount of time. Over time the $25 will become irrelevant to how you live your life. The $25 will have no bearing on what you spend for groceries, how you pay your utilities, or even how or what you choose as recreation. This same idea applies to goals about health and fitness – it's baby steps. In essence, when we set healthy eating as a goal, the changes we make in what we eat should be minimal enough at each stage to become irrelevant to how we live our lives. If we can accomplish this, there's no perceptible disruption to our eating lifestyle, and therefore little to no resistance to overcome. So to set effective goals: 1) make them small and 2) keep them free from time constraints. If you can do this, making lifestyle or diet changes to reach your goals will be much easier! The changes are subtle so we barely realize the change is occurring, and we have no time pressure because we are in no hurry. We can take as much time as we want to implement subtle changes in our behavior.

Implementing Dietary Baby-Steps

Let's say you are sitting down watching television and eating your favorite (and unhealthy) meal: a cheeseburger, fries and a soda. All you have to do to make a subtle change is to eliminate a small portion of the soft drink. That's it! Enjoy the rest. Then once you are used to eating this meal with the reduced portion of soda, eliminate a small portion of the fries. I use the term *eliminate* because this part of your meal has to be physically removed, so throw it in the garbage or pour it down the sink. If we do not completely eliminate the portions we are subtracting from our meal then we have the opportunity to go back and consume them. Get rid of it.

As we continuously eliminate portions of our unhealthy meal, then we should add in something healthy to replace what's missing and keep the portion size the same. We don't want to starve the body by cutting portion size at this point. There is no reason to rush the process. We have all the time in the world to succeed. By taking our time, we inscribe these modifications as a forever change, not a temporary fad or passing phase. The subtlety of the changes means you will not experience periods of withdrawal mentally or physically, and your taste buds and mind won't be alerted to reject the healthy substitutions. When we implement healthy choices too quickly, then the food we are trying to eliminate becomes a huge monster. And if we make the things we love to eat and drink into enemies, then our minds will prepare for battle. And as you probably know because you are reading this book, going into a diet or weight-loss program with a battle mentality ensures resistance that often leads to failure. Baby steps are non-threatening, gradual, and lead to bigger strides and later success.

Subtle changes are barely noticed by the eye, so they're less likely to be noticed by the mind. For instance, if you had a jar of pennies and I took one penny out of the jar each day, it would be some time before you realized the pennies were missing. And by the time your mind realizes those pennies were going away, it's too late - they're already gone. This is how we have to play the food game. By the time your mind and body realize a particular food has gone away, it should be too late. Once one item of the meal which we are attempting to change is partially eliminated we move to the next item of food. Don't fall into the trap of sequential elimination if your favorite food is part of a "set" or meal. So continuing the example of the fast food meal, we don't completely eliminate the soft drink before we start working on the burger or the fries. This is because water does not taste good with burgers and fries at this stage in the game. So what happens is we increase the likelihood of re-instituting the soft drink into the meal rather than drinking the decreased amount of soft drink during the meal. So we treat the whole meal in the same manner. We can't eliminate the entire box of fries from the meal and think this is going to stick. The likelihood of picking up some or all of those fries to include with this meal becomes greater.

Another potential trap we may set for ourselves is to buy a smaller or kid size meal instead of buying the normal or supersized meal we are used to. This substitution does not have the same effect as the slow elimination, so stick with the same sized meal you would normally purchase. At some point in eliminating portions of the normal sized meal we have a conscious thought of money being wasted. The money being wasted serves a couple of purposes. First, we're throwing away money by wasting food. We can use this as motivation - but only if we plan to use this money for something good and positive. Secondly, when we throw away part of this meal and replace it with something healthy, we are practicing making conscious decisions about food choices. For example, I might as well fill the rest of the unhealthy meal with the healthy foods I am slowly implementing.   Your ability to sustain this behavior is much greater when you add it gradually, rather than going cold turkey. Moreover, reinstituting the unhealthy food should eventually cause a negative reaction in your body. For example, the grease from the burger may cause you to have stomach pains, indigestion, or other symptoms because your body no longer wants the unhealthy food products.

Tips for Travelers

We have talked about how to slowly eliminate unhealthy eating within our own homes. For some, traveling for work or business may mean that dining out -- and fast food -- is a part of the weekly routine. I am always trying to come up with new ways to help motivate my clients when they are traveling, because I know it is very difficult to eat healthy on the road. If you travel for business you are probably used to grabbing fast food or a quick bite in between sales call, or having meetings over a big, calorie-dense lunch or dinner. So how do we implement the same principles of eliminating unhealthy eating when we travel? In the same slow manner we would at home – we just have to be a bit more creative, and keep in mind that it will still be a slow process. Any change is better than no change at all.

One suggestion is to get into the habit of taking healthy food items with you on your travels – in the car or in your carry-on bag. Protein bars, fruit, almonds, and other quick healthy snacks can be eaten on the go. Having these snacks with you and accessible, especially if you are driving, gives you the opportunity to grab something out of a cooler and eat it while you're traveling, instead of getting hungry and stopping for fast food. If in the beginning of your dietary change fast food is your main staple while traveling, don't eliminate going through the drive through. Instead, order what you normally would, and then when you pick it up, pull up next to the trash can and take some of the fries and throw them out, and/or pour out some of the soda. Make these actions a habit, and then build on these actions the same way you would if you were sitting in front of your television. So if you throw out part of the meal you just purchased, what do you replace it with? The healthy snack you have packed away in your bag or cooler.

If you are at a sit-down restaurant taking a meeting, order something healthier than other products on the menu. Then, before your meal hits the table -- and this includes any bread, chips or salad -- drink two full glasses of water. Make sure it's bottled water because it should be cleaner than the tap water they bring you in a glass full of ice. The water you drink before your meal arrives causes your stomach to be full ahead of time, and therefore you should not be able to eat as much of the food on your plate. This works the same for alcoholic beverages: drink large amounts of water before you start drinking alcoholic beverages and you'll consume less alcohol, which contains large amounts of calories per volume.

Substituting with Food Substitutes?

Often when I discuss this idea of preventing a battle against favorite foods, my clients ask whether they can just switch their full calorie version to diet, sugar-free, or fat-free versions. In my opinion, adding so-called "diet" foods to replace the unhealthier foods you love to eat is completely wrong. Labeling aside, the fact that we are trying to find a substitute for a meal or favorite food means we are not making healthy changes as describe above. Eating diet or reduced fat ice cream does not change the way the mind thinks about ice cream. Drinking a diet soft drink does not change the way the mind thinks about the soft drink and, in a pinch, you won't grab the diet soft drink anyway. In any case, if you compare the labels between "regular" and "diet" versions of a particular food, you are likely to find the difference between the two is very subtle. And typically natural ingredients are replaced with chemicals and synthetics that have been created to eliminate calories. Moreover, the slight differences in actual ingredients are overlaid with marketing designs and messages developed precisely to make you feel like this is a better or healthier choice. Remember, the company that makes this diet product is in the business of making money, not in the business of helping you to lose weight. This means your health and fitness are not their bottom line or ultimate goal. The bottom line is revenue generated from sales of this product. This alone should anger you enough to avoid dietary food products as a way to lose weight. View this as a negative situation which motivates you into a positive choice or action: to eliminate portions of the unhealthy food product until you reach your goal of eliminating it all together.

A Few Words about Carbs

When we are forming new, healthy eating habits, it often seems carbohydrates are a food source we try to eliminate. This makes sense because complex carbohydrates like white rice and potatoes, pasta, and bread are foods which quickly turn into sugars in the body. These carbohydrate sugars turn into fat faster than any other food product we can take in; carbohydrates go into our fatty storage cells if our metabolism is unable to burn them off. But from my experience as a personal trainer and a bodybuilder, I know how drastically reducing carbohydrates in the diet can cause mood swings. One client whom I put on a reduced carbohydrate food plan became testier towards the workout regimen as the level of carbohydrates decreased. This client -- a very nice person -- experienced negative mood changes and mood swings during our sessions because of the low level of complex carbohydrates he was taking in. This has happened with both male and female clients.

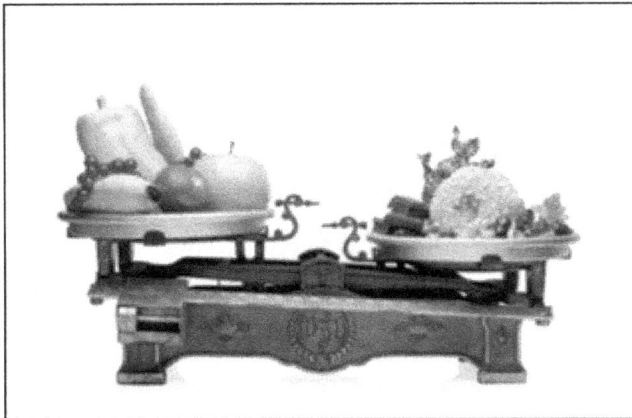

One of the ways to help prevent the mood swings of lowering carbohydrates while changing food habits is to eat the major portions of carbohydrates in the morning as your first meal. When you wake up in the morning your body is basically empty because it has metabolized all of the food that you ate the previous night. This means the digestive system, metabolism and fatty stores have completed their task. When you wake in the morning, your body is prepared to be fueled and can metabolize a higher level of complex carbohydrates than it can later in the day. I'm sure you've heard that breakfast is the most important meal of the day. That expression is absolutely true in terms of how we fuel our bodies and how we metabolize complex carbohydrates.

When you eat your major complex carbohydrate meal as the first meal, you should then consume carbohydrates in moderation each meal thereafter. If you are the type of person who loves to eat big pasta meals at lunch or dinner, and you enjoy a second helping, you're going to have to practice moderation. Motivate yourself to eat moderately, and be conscious of your body's signals of satiety. Our stomachs are actually full 15 minutes prior to the brain sending the signal that we are full. This means there is no need for the second helping. The second helping during the meal takes a body from full to stuffed, and we know what happens when we're stuffed: we get tired, we get the lethargic, and we want to lie down and rest. I call this after-dinner hibernation. After-dinner hibernation goes like this: you get up from the table, sit down on the couch, pull up a blanket, click on the television, and usually fall asleep for a postprandial nap in order to digest the meal you have eaten. If you eat the majority of your complex carbohydrates early in the day and only in moderation after that, you can avoid the hibernation effect – and the effects it has on your body and weight.

Carrying the Changes Forward

The steps you take to decrease the amount of unhealthy food you consume on a daily basis should serve as motivation to continue forward. Use your small successes in order to feel proud of what you've accomplished. Mentally reward yourself every time you make a positive or healthy choice. Use these moments to recognize you have accomplished a small goal, you have moved one step forward, and reward yourself with happiness. The happiness you feel and the pride you take from crossing the small hurdles will allow you to build momentum on your journey to completion of the bigger goals. The momentum that you gain by making these small changes, by working on changing your habits, will increase as you push forward in eliminating your unhealthy eating. This momentum will lead you to being on the other end of the healthy/unhealthy eating scale, to the point where three quarters of any given meal is healthy.

When you reach the point where healthy eating outweighs unhealthy eating, your taste buds will have adapted to the healthier offerings. This should lead to better enjoyment of the natural organic flavors in fruits, vegetables, and meats that are untainted by industry. Like many of my clients, I have also implemented juicing of fruits and vegetables into my daily food planning, and the funny thing is my taste buds have adapted to the natural earthy taste of juicing. When I first started juicing, just like most of my clients, I remember the juice tasting like dirt. Many of my clients complain to me about the same issue, but now I have a completely different outlook when I'm drinking down 10 or 12 ounces of organic juice. The earthier the taste to the juice, the better my understanding of its chemical-free nature. Not putting chemicals in your body should make you feel a sense of renewal and peace about how you are treating your body. That said, I do not recommend vegetarianism or vegan diets, because, in my opinion, any form of vegetarianism is an incomplete way of fueling the human body. We have developed and evolved canine teeth for a reason, and that, in my opinion, is to consume a certain amount of meat.

Implementing a Ketosis Day

So now you've switched from unhealthy eating to healthy eating and you have done it in a way which did not destroy your life or lifestyle. The healthy eating is dominating your meals without the sense of being stressed because you have to record every meal and count calories because you have done it the slow, natural way. Is this the end of the journey? Do you continue this for the rest of your life? The answer is no. Once you have reached your goal weight, and even during the process of losing weight, I don't believe every single meal, every single day, should be healthy or clean. As I mentioned in the previous chapter, implement a ketosis or "cheat" day once a week where you get to eat one or two meals of whatever you would like. I prefer to call it a *ketosis* day rather than *cheat* day because of the negative connotation surrounding the word *cheat*. Cheating is not something we're proud of or want to be associated with, and when it comes to our diet, we do want to be proud.

Incorporating a ketosis day into your routine generates a few different effects in your mind. The first is a recognition that you can still eat processed, unnatural, unhealthy type foods, but only for one day per week. So again, the idea of going cold turkey or never having some of your favorite food products is less, and resistance to the change is eliminated. The next reason for having one day a week to eat a couple meals of whatever you want is the physiological process of ketosis. Think of ketosis as the human body's way of adjusting for the excess fats and sugars of the "cheat" day. I like to call the ketosis process a panic mode for your metabolism. When you eat clean for six days and then on the seventh day eat one or two unhealthy meals, your metabolism realizes the change and it speeds up for two or three days thereafter to compensate and to burn off the extra carbohydrates and fats and sugars. For some people, going through ketosis causes them to actually lose more weight during this process. Moreover, the weight that is being lost during the ketosis process is usually more fat than water. When I was competing as a bodybuilder, it was during this time of ketosis that I would notice huge changes in my physique.

During the ketosis day, my advice is to try not to treat it as a free-for-all. I have done this before and wouldn't do it again. In my experience, when you eat clean six days and then choose to gorge yourself on unhealthy food on the seventh day, you can become very ill. This is another reason I advocate a ketosis day. Juxtaposing how we feel after eating clean for six days and then how we feel after eating our old favorites helps us to realize our sensitivity to chemically-based foods. I have many clients who tell me the ketosis day isn't as satisfying as what they would have thought because of the feeling of nausea, gas, or indigestion from eating heavy chemically-based foods. So we may be able to use the effects of eating unhealthy foods on our ketosis day as a motivation to eat slightly cleaner even on the ketosis day. What I mean by this is instead of eating a burger from a fast food restaurant, grill your own burger. Instead of eating ice cream from the supermarket, go out to an ice cream parlor or get it fresh or from a gourmet ice cream shop. So even though you are having your ketosis day, you are eating it in a more natural and healthy way, reducing the amount of chemicals and other "processing" ingredients you ingest. You will still have the benefits from sending your body into ketosis, and can help you realize how far your eating choices – and your control over those choices – have progressed. The ketosis day reminds us we are going through a series of changes, and it reminds us both mentally and physically of where we were and how far we have come.

Keeping the Fire Burning

Despite the smallness of the changes you're making to your diet, the changes that you will see and feel are huge. Your body is an organic machine, and when you fuel it with good quality fuel, you get improved performance in all aspects of being. Think about putting wood on a fire to heat your home. What good would it be to open the furnace door and throw wet wood on the fire? The fire can only smolder and smoke - it cannot reach its maximum heating potential. On the other hand, when you are using good, hard, cured wood to heat your furnace, that fire is going to burn hot. In the same way, when you fill your body with good, healthy, organic foods, your metabolism speeds up, burning fat more efficiently to help shed the pounds even faster. Keep with it, and feel good about the changes you are making.

Chapter 5: But Don't I Need a Personal Trainer?

With changes in diet underway, using the baby steps approach, you can add in daily movement, exercise, or workouts to help burn calories, increase your cardiovascular fitness, and tone and sculpt your muscles. In the previous chapters, I have talked about different forms of motivation. And as a person looking to get motivated to lose weight, you should ask yourself, "Can I motivate myself? If I cannot afford a personal trainer can I still get the job done?" Some people – those who are motivated by something or have completely made a decision to motivate themselves -- can use this motivation to get to a point where they're making good decisions about their eating habits, losing weight, and reaching their goals. On the other hand, there are people looking to lose weight who are not in a particular state of mind to motivate themselves. The question is, *Do you need a personal trainer to motivate you?* I can't answer that question for you, just as I can't take your journey to health and fitness for you. But I can tell you this: You can lose weight without a personal trainer. In this chapter, I'll give you tips on how to succeed in self-motivating to add exercise into your weight loss plan. If you think you need a personal trainer to guide you toward your goals, I encourage you to read the next few chapters, and then assess again. If you still believe you need a personal trainer, Chapter 9 outlines some criteria to help you select a good one.

You Can 'Do It Yourself'

Self-motivating can be very difficult. We live in a society that is increasingly dependent or needy. This manifests in the realm of health and fitness as the belief that we have to hire a personal trainer and go to a gym in order to accomplish our health goals. But personal trainers are just another tool to assist you in your weight loss; hiring a personal trainer does not determine whether you're going to lose weight or reach your goals. I know a lot of personal trainers with obese clients. These clients start a weight loss process, and after they lose five or 10 pounds, the trainer sets them loose. Those clients are still obese. I know personal trainers working with clients to get them stronger too. These clients end up gaining weight because of the muscles they build, and in the grand scheme of things, this is a positive development because muscle burns more calories than fat. But the clients cannot control what they are doing outside of the gym -- self-motivating to change their diets - so they do not lose any weight. So it is very possible to NOT lose weight with a personal trainer. The good news is that the inverse is also true: you CAN lose weight without a personal trainer. If you structure the way you make changes in your life properly, you can do the job of losing weight and getting fit yourself.

To do this, you will have to understand certain aspects of fitness and nutrition. Given the public health crisis of obesity in our society, there are enormous amounts of information on shedding pounds available to you – on the Internet and in libraries and bookstores -- that you should take full advantage of. Gather resources and information about the human body, food plans, workouts, training regimens, and dietary supplements to help you work towards reaching your fitness goals. I also recommend looking in the self-help section of the bookstore to see what speaks to you. This can help you change your mind about other negative habits in your life so there is a complete metamorphosis, not just of the body but of the mind as well. This is what ultimately determines your success – how far you can go to alter your mind. This is why personal trainers do not guarantee weight loss, because they cannot live in your head. What can guarantee that you reach your goal is altering your state of mind so that you think differently about health and fitness, about your weight loss. Even better, eventually you will not have to think about it at all. Health and fitness, a good diet, and regular exercise can and will become second nature, just like waking up and brushing your teeth.

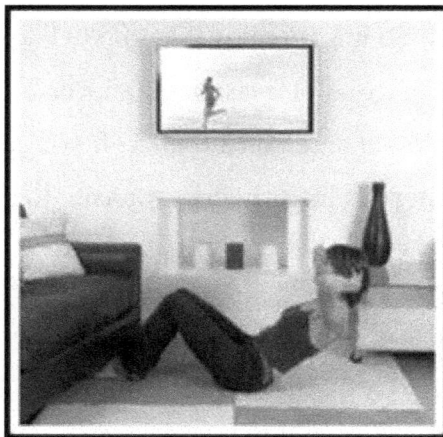

You Can Do It at Home

As we think about health and fitness being second nature, let's also consider the necessity of a gym or fitness facility to reach our fitness goals. As with the 'need' for a personal trainer, there is no *need* to pay a monthly fee to enter a place where there is equipment, other people, or sometimes distractions in order to reach our fitness goals and become healthier people. Just being active and doing more than you did on your way to gaining the weight will start the process of shedding pounds and reversing obesity. So if you do not have a gym or fitness facility, what do you do or where do you go for exercise? There are plenty of options in your own home, like a spare bedroom, basement, or garage. Find a spot where you can lay out a couple of mats, put up a small television, get a few free weights, and some workout videos. Add some fresh plants and make sure you have nice lighting and upbeat colors to make it an inviting personal workout space. Over time, setting up your own workout space will cost you considerably less than the gym membership that you would be paying for even when you're not going to the gym. You can also go outside in the sunshine and nature to get some vitamin D and fresh air. In the spring, summer, and fall your training may happen at a park or lake or some other outdoor venue. In the winter this may be a little bit more difficult, but you will have your personal workout space to retreat to, where you can continue to stretch, do push-ups, sit-ups and free squats in order to keep your body in motion to burn fat and continue weight loss. None of these suggestions requires you going to a fitness facility. They don't require you to give anyone money to become healthy. That said, many people already have a gym membership, and find they enjoy the social scene of at least seeing other people working out around them, if not talking to them and striking up conversations. If you think that sounds like you, I'll give you some tips for making the most of your gym time in Chapter 7. In either case, you will need to build a resistance to the negative voices in your head and create within yourself the aptitude for self-motivation. This means you will have to take on the burden of being able to motivate yourself. In essence you will have to become your own personal trainer.

Becoming Your Own Personal Trainer

Is self-motivation more difficult than being motivated by someone like a personal trainer? The answer for most is *yes,* but that does not mean it's impossible. And when you get the hang of it, it's so much more effective. So how do we go about creating motivation to train ourselves? My clients always tell me they get better workouts with me than what they would do themselves. I personally do not get better workouts when someone else is training me. I actually get better workouts pushing myself from within my own head, listening to the personal trainer within my mind. There is always a part of you which is telling you not to quit. Are you listening? If you have chosen to work out in your own workout space and to be your own personal trainer, are you willing to listen to that alter ego? If you can develop the will, strength, and fortitude of mind to know how to listen to your own voice saying, "One more rep, one more set," then you can be your own personal trainer.

When a person develops the ability to start self-motivating in small ways to change habits, there are going to be obstacles to appraise, tackle, and overcome. One of the first challenges is to develop partial willpower. I say partial willpower because complete willpower seems to cause people who are trying to lose weight to go in the opposite direction. Losing weight is not always about willpower. There are other factors in people's lives dictating eating habits which lead to weight gain and obesity. Sometimes people are emotional eaters, so when there are stressors in life that they are unable to deal with directly, it manifests itself in a type of eating disorder. People like this feel they are not in control of how much food they eat, how frequently they eat, and/or what they eat. I do not believe this is a sign of weakness or a lack of willpower. What it signals to me is that this person needs to change – mentally as much as or more than physically. When we realize we have to change the way we think, how we view ourselves in health and fitness, then we are taking one of the baby steps towards success.

This change in self-perception relates directly to how you become your own personal trainer. You have to step outside of your normal perspective and be able to look at yourself from an elevated position, a position of understanding, and work from there. When you look in the mirror and you are observing your body or thinking about your eating habits, your fitness level, and other things that affect the way you look and feel about yourself, you have to do it in a way of non-judgmental self-assessment. You need a baseline before you implement change, and benchmarks along the way. During this assessment process in your mind, use a neutral lens. Remove the negativity and judgment; don't stand in front of the mirror and beat yourself up because of what you see. During this assessment, create an image in your mind of what you would *like* to see in the future. Embrace this image you now see in your mind. Smile and say, "I am motivated by what I see."

This does two things: First, you have created an image in your mind of where you would like to see yourself and you are saying you are motivated by where you would like to be. You are motivating yourself by envisioning the future you. Second, as you're looking at yourself in the mirror, you have a physical image of yourself and you are saying, "I am motivated by what I see at this point." You are being motivated by the unhealthy person who is out of shape and has bad habits, someone who isn't working out. You are not judging that person, you are simply positively motivated by the negatives you perceive. What we have done is to take a completely negative image and put a positive spin on it. This means that you do not have to speak negatively about the image of the person you presently see in the mirror.

If you are obese – or even just carrying an extra 10-15 pounds – the image of your body you see in the mirror should still be treated with respect. We should never say things like *I'm fat* or *I'm disgusting* or *I hate myself.* When we think about self-motivation, we have to look at the negative and flip it to view the positive side so we don't undermine our potential for success. Thinking this way does not mean we accept what we see in the mirror and say it's okay to be 30, 75 or 100 pounds overweight. This way of thinking is negative motivation. Of course you are beautiful inside, but that does not mean you have to carry an extra 100 pounds. What I mean is that if you are successful in business or a great mother or has amazing people skills; don't accept obesity as part of your success and accomplishments. Hold yourself accountable for the things that deep down inside you feel are out of your control. Do not get into the habit of wrapping your obesity and your poor eating habits and lack of exercise in a pretty bow and calling it powerful, or proud, or whatever word you want to call it in order to avoid answering to yourself the way you should. Do something about it.

The self-assessment is a first step in accepting responsibility for what currently is. Don't be afraid of what comes out of the self-assessment. We self-assess at different points in our day, in our week, in the month, and the year. Self-assessment is a natural process in our lives. Obesity or weight gain doesn't happen overnight. It is for most a very slow process, and during this process there was undoubtedly self-assessment going on. A weight gain of

50 pounds happens in small increments. During these small increments of weight gain we see ourselves in the mirror after a shower and we self-assess. When one of our loving children says in their childish honesty, "Mommy/Daddy, you are fat," we self-assess. During this self-assessment we understand that over the past year we've gained 10 pounds. We know in our minds and in our hearts that if we do not change our negative habits we are going to gain another five or 10 pounds over the next year. We know this. It is not a surprise. People pretend weight gain is a complete surprise and act like they woke up this morning 50 pounds overweight. The surprise should be the lack of action or response while you were inching up to 50 extra pounds.

Whether you are 15 or 50 or 150 pounds overweight, you must have self-assessed in some form or another many different times during the slow weight gain. Often during the self-assessment we lie to ourselves and say, *Well it's 5 pounds, I can lose the weight in a week* or *My New Year's resolution is to lose the 10 pounds that I gained this year.* We tell ourselves small white lies in order to justify or ignore our weight gain. Of course, weight gain is gradual because the body does not want to be obese or to carry extra weight so it is always fighting to be at your natural weight for the age that you are right now. If we woke up and suddenly we were obese, it would probably take the same amount of time to lose the weight – basically overnight. So why would we think it should take a short amount of time to lose weight when it took a long amount of time to gain weight? What I'm saying here is keep things in perspective. If we keep our weight loss and our weight loss motivation in perspective, then we do not have to little-white-lie ourselves out of reaching our goals. We do not have to little-white-lie ourselves into creating reasons why we cannot succeed in reaching our weight loss goals.

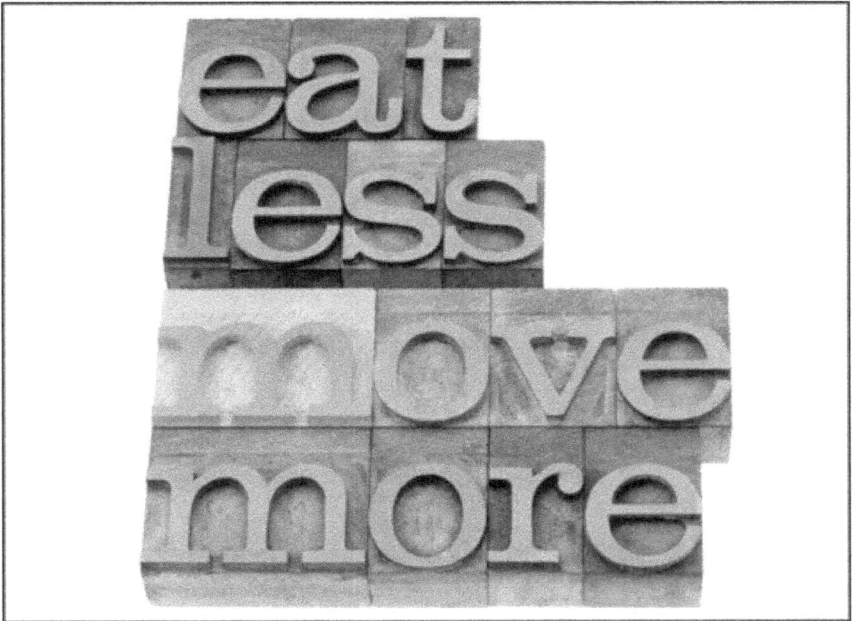

Little White Lies

Let's talk a little bit more about the little white lies we tell ourselves to give us the out, to talk ourselves into being okay with being heavy or to justify our absences from the gym. These little white lies hold us back from creating a healthy and fit body. So how do we take this way of thinking and change it? This is where we use your internal personal trainer. Stop telling yourself you are happy the way you are; expect more of yourself. Use the personal trainer you are developing within to squash the little white lies, including the lie that you are happy with who you are if you are fat. There is nothing happy about being fat or obese and not being able to control your eating habits or weight. If you are truly happy, I guarantee you would be happier if you lost the weight, because no one wants to carry around an extra 50 or 100 pounds everywhere they go. I know this because if you gave a person who is fit an extra 50 or 100 pounds to carry around everywhere they went, they would be very unhappy. Saying you are happy with who you are or happy with being heavy is a copout, and since we're talking about little white lies, I'm going to call you out on it bluntly. I know you would be happier not carrying the extra weight around because not only is the weight a physical burden, but it exposes you to prejudice every day of your life. And being judged (negatively) everywhere you go about the way you look cannot make anyone happy. It's a fact of life in our society that there are prejudices about people who are overweight. They are considered lazy, greedy, weak, and/or lacking willpower or self-control. People do not look at fat people and say to themselves, "I know she's beautiful inside." As human beings, our reactions to visual stimuli are thoughts that appraise or judge the form, without an immediate filter of political correctness. So I'm not going to talk about obesity in a politically correct way. I'm not going to mince words in order to save you a little embarrassment, because my goal is to encourage you to be accountable for your negative or unhealthy habits.

So now that we've dispensed with the use of little white lies to accept our extra weight, let's discuss how we can use the little white lies for motivation. If we return to the idea of self-assessment, we can use our imaginations to envision the fitter and leaner self we desire, and then we can create and write down some little white lies to help us with the process. For example, if you envision the way your face will look without excess weight, you might say, *I love my beautiful, pronounced cheekbones.* It is a little white lie, but one that can motivate us into creating a positive self-image. It's a projection of where we are going. Those little white lies are a forecast of the end of your journey, and they are important because they start the process of changing the mind. Telling yourself you are beautiful during your assessment because you can see a slender person who is not obese in your mind's eye creates a positive change.

These little white lies can help create a detailed positive image that, once created, can lead to more positive thoughts. Let's say you are imagining your arms are smaller, your face is more sculpted, your thighs are thinner, and then you can imagine the smaller person within. If you can imagine the person within as a stronger person, you will become stronger. We become what we imagine; we will become what our mind's eye sees. This is a great strategy to use even before setting goals because during the journey this is exactly what's happening. As you are losing weight you are becoming stronger. The simple fact that you are exercising will help to compact the bones in your body which will make your bone density stronger. Not having to carry around the extra weight will make you more flexible, more mobile, and even faster. Telling yourself this ahead of time, before it actually happens, allows you to create that positive foundation we discussed earlier. Moreover, your mind will become stronger. At the end of your journey when your body is stronger, you are carrying around less weight, your muscles are showing, and your body is sculpted, your mind will be stronger. This can be for many people a complete transformation of a former self. Imagine you are the caterpillar who is beautiful -- fat and chunky-- but still beautiful. The caterpillar is carrying more weight in order to make it through its metamorphosis in the cocoon. That caterpillar then emerges as a lightweight, sleek butterfly. The butterfly that was once the caterpillar shows a significant change and so will you.

Give It Time

As we think about a butterfly emerging from a cocoon, we know it took time for the journey the caterpillar had to take inside of that cocoon. The manifestation of the butterfly does not occur in a moment. Similarly, our metamorphosis is going to take time. During our transformation we are going to have to make changes in very small increments in what we do during our day. If there are bad habits you have, they should be changed in the slightest manner so the change can almost not be seen, felt, heard, or tasted.

Let's return to an example from our plan to make dietary changes. If you are sitting in front of the TV and eating a burger and fries and drinking a soft drink, you are not moving around. If you are not moving around, your metabolism is likely slowing down. So if one of the things causing you to be obese is sitting down to watch television, change it. Change the negative habit and replace it with positive things that will become positive habits. But remember, we're not trying to make drastic changes. So instead of turning off the television and getting up and trying to run a mile, start by turning off the television for an hour and reading a book. If you're sitting in the same chair reading a book on health and fitness rather than watching TV, your metabolism will not likely speed up. But you've eliminated an hour's worth of ads that could possibly lead to unhealthy eating and replaced it with knowledge about something healthier for you. The next step, once your mind gets used to reading a book instead of watching television is to add movement.

Go take a walk. Don't think of it as exercise, just getting out stretching your legs and seeing what's going on in the world. Obviously what we're talking about again here is taking baby steps. Because these steps are more psychological than physical, you do not need a personal trainer for this process. And actually, most personal trainers would probably not have the knowledge to even set you on this path.

Chapter 6: Money Saved is Fit Spendable

Another way to motivate and reward yourself for being your own personal trainer is to keep track of the money you would have been spending on a professional trainer and put it toward achieving your fitness goals on your own. The cost of personal training may run from $15 to $90 or more for a half-hour session. Calculate what a personal trainer would cost you per session, and put that amount in a jar or separate bank account each time you successfully train yourself. For example, if a personal trainer will cost $35 per session, pay yourself $35 per session to work out on your own. The money you get from personal training yourself and motivating yourself will increase with every workout you have. So with every session you train yourself, pay yourself. Don't skimp! A personal trainer expects payment for every session and so should you. After just 40 sessions at $35 each, you will have paid *yourself* $1400 that you can use to help educate yourself, purchase workout equipment, or simply reward yourself with a nice little trip to enjoy the new leaner, stronger you! This is what I'm talking about when I say that money saved it fit spendable.

Make the Most of Your Hard-Earned Cash

If you calculate that you'll save thousands of dollars by training yourself, you might decide to go out immediately and buy a complete home gym to help with your self-training. **Big mistake!** I say that for two reasons. First, you haven't earned that money yet. You have to be the trainer you are paying yourself to be, each and every session for that 10 or 12 week period, before you will have earned that money. Secondly, if you buy a new home gym or a room full of equipment in your first week, the motivational effect of both the cash incentive and the equipment will be short lived. You can only spend as much on health and fitness as you've earned by working out and training yourself, so think about incremental purchases that will both motivate you and keep your workouts fresh. For example, a fitness mat is a good first purchase. You can get a decent one for around $25, so you will still have extra cash to put away toward whatever reward or larger purchase you have set as a longer-term goal. Put the mat in your workout room, or an area where you can use it to do a simple but effective workout. Start with push-ups, sit-ups, and free squats. These exercises are about all you need when you are at the very beginning of your fitness journey. Think about doing just three sets of 10 reps of each exercise. If that proves to be too difficult, back it up to 8 or 5 reps. Remember, baby steps and incremental progress will get you there more effectively than over-reaching. Keep doing those particular exercises until you are able to accomplish the full three sets, so 30 repetitions per exercise. At this point, you have reached your first small goal.

Once you have accomplished this first step (and have earned some additional cash for training yourself to reach that goal),reward yourself by purchasing a stability ball, a medicine ball, or a pair of 5 or 10 pound dumbbells -- but nothing more. You see where this is going, right? As we increase our fitness level, we increase the tools we have available to create different workouts. By adding equipment in this piecemeal fashion, we get little gifts to commemorate our achievements, motivate us to keep going, and to add something new and interesting to our workouts. Each new piece of equipment will expand the range of exercises and movements you can do to strengthen your body, and will give an added boost of encouragement to your mind. During this process you are not spending any "extra" money because you are your own personal trainer; the money you are using for equipment is part of the money you would be using to pay personal trainer. But instead, you are the owner, operator, personal trainer, and client of your own gradually expanding gym. If you are using an existing gym, come up with some similarly small, incremental rewards for your progress. These may be clothes or accessories to highlight your changing body or small trips to the beach or mountains or someplace you find inspiration. The underlying principles of rewarding yourself for "good behavior" are the same.

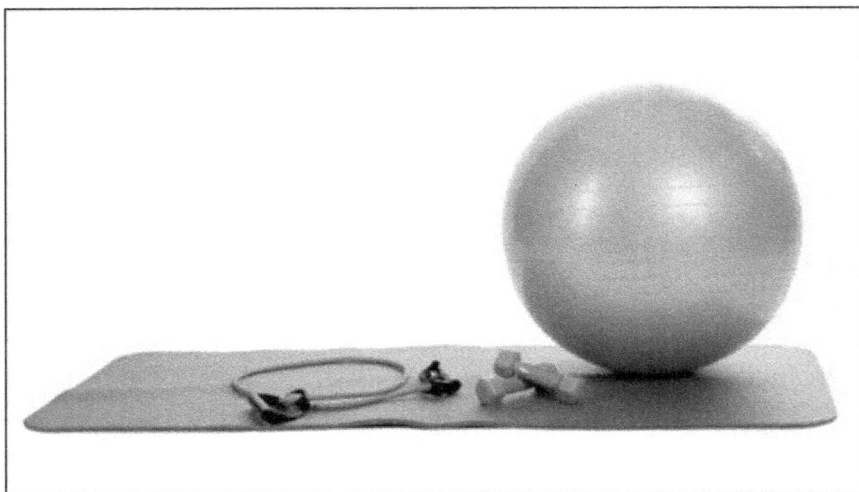

Make the Most of Your Equipment

If you have started purchasing fitness equipment to reward yourself for becoming stronger – or if you're working out in one small section of the gym – you'll next need to start thinking about the range of goals you can set for yourself with each piece of equipment. For example, if you have already reached your goal of 30 reps of push-ups, sit-ups, and squats, what's next? Increase the sets or reps? No. There's not enough muscle confusion in these kinds of goals to keep your body guessing as to what and how it will be expected to perform. Instead, think about how you can modify the exercise or use the equipment differently. For our example, you can do the same exercises in a different way by changing your body position, like the distance between your feet or hands. So if you're in a push-up position and your hands are directly below or beneath your shoulders, spread your hands out on the floor 6 inches further than your shoulders. If you are doing front squats with feet directly beneath your shoulders, move your feet 6 inches past your shoulders and squat from there. Changing your position works in the opposite direction as well. Moving your hands or feet closer together or toward the center of your body is also very effective. There should be an element of creativity in your workouts and in your exercises no matter what equipment you have or don't have.

Finally, related to both body position and equipment, a crucial element to remember is proper form. As you get started with your own personal training, you should always be correcting your form (so a mirror may be one of the first pieces of equipment you buy with your fitness savings). One of your goals for every workout should be to have correct form in every exercise you do. You will have to be vigilant in reminding yourself to use proper form since you are client and trainer. This will help to prevent injuries later on, when you work up to purchasing and using larger and heavier weights. They say old habits die hard, but if we establish good habits from the beginning -- good posture, good form, correct lifting -- there will be fewer bad habits to contend with later on.

Chapter 7: I Just Don't Feel Like It Today

You have been training yourself. You have been slowly changing your diet. The hard work is paying off in the form of improved energy, stronger muscles; less fat... and then one day you wake up and just don't feel like doing it. Any of it. Maybe you haven't had enough sleep. Maybe you're stressed about work or the holidays or any number of things. Or maybe you are just so *bored* with all of it. There are many reasons to incorporate variety, flexibility, and creativity into your workout schedule, but the ability to maintain a consistent commitment to working out while listening and responding to your body are among the most important. And this leads us to the question of how to keep things interesting.

How do I keep my workouts fresh and exciting?

It's very common to get stuck in a rut when we're working out. We pick our favorite exercises, our favorite pieces of equipment, and our favorite days to work out and before we know it, three months have gone by and we're still doing the same workout as when we started. No wonder we're bored! Workouts become exciting when there's a new element or challenge. Simply adding a different machine, exercise or piece of equipment to your workout will engage your body and mind in something novel, forcing it to pay attention and not rely on muscle memory. Mixing things up on a regular basis also ensures your muscles are making larger gains during the exercise process, because they don't become over-efficient at any one motion or movement.

Rainy & Sunny Day Workouts

Once you embrace the benefits of diverse workouts, be sure to tune in to how your body feels on a given day. How do you feel when you wake up in the morning and the sky is overcast or it's raining outside? For most everyone I know, gray or rainy weather inspires desires to pull on a blanket and sit on the couch with a movie or book rather than going out for a run or to the gym. So there is what I call a rainy day workout and a sunny day workout. And your body responds to each very differently. In the rainy day state of mind, your workout cannot and should not be the same as when the sun is out. When it is raining and you are trying to get to the gym and have a workout, there are changes in physical characteristics of your muscles and joints that could make you more susceptible to injury if you do your "normal" workout routine. It will take longer for your muscles to warm up and your joints to get loosened up in preparation for good workouts. So if you have a schedule, if your workout is planned and you have no flexibility to change it, you could be facing a nagging injury in your future. Moreover, your mind may not be completely involved in the exercise you're doing if at this point you've dragged yourself out of bed to get to the gym in the first place.

The sunny day workout allows you to capitalize on good feelings and the "excitement of growth" to push yourself to the next level. Science has shown us that we respond, in terms of our moods and energy, to sunlight: our energy and state of mind change when the sun is out. So let's say the sun is out, the weather is warm, and you go to the gym. You are excited about your workout, and you are probably feeling good, happy, and strong. If at this point you pull out a schedule or workout plan with an outline that shows you're going to be doing the exact same thing you did yesterday or two days ago, where's the fun in that? Where's the excitement in being able to utilize the energy you received from the sun being out. Some of the best workouts I have had were when the sun was out.

There is no reason to treat one workout the same as any other. Working out should be fun first and foremost. If you are not having fun and doing a workout or going to the gym feels like going to a second job, it's pretty likely that you will not participate for long. It has to be fun!

Ask for help

If you are working out at a gym, asking someone to give you assistance during an exercise is an excellent way to add a new dimension to your workout. Having someone else involved creates an element of excitement because most people do not like to ask other people in the gym to give them a spot. When you are trying to push yourself a little bit harder than normal in the gym, ask someone to assist you. When you do this the other person usually has a different perspective on the exercise you are doing, so it can be a great way to learn things. You might also strike up a conversation about health and fitness in general, and find out some tips or tricks that have helped someone else, that you could incorporate into your own journey to keep it moving along. I have learned a great deal of information by asking for assistance during a workout. Some of the information I have gained I used for my own workouts and some I set aside because it was not right for the type of fitness journey I was on at the time. Additionally, when you gain new perspective about exercises or fitness in general, and then implement them into your own workout regimen, it will help to keep your muscles confused, thus giving you a greater workout.

Just the experience of interacting with someone else can turn out to be refreshing and add a social element to the workout experience. Asking someone for a spot or assistance can also serve as a great icebreaker. In my experience, in gyms where members think this way, it becomes infectious and the next thing you know, just about everybody knows everybody. (Of course this works better in a smaller gym than a large corporate gym.) If you really want to change the energy of your workout, try observing a few people who are on your same level and approach them about getting together for a group workout. Working out in groups creates a different dynamic and energizes the workout session. It's like taking a fitness class, except there is no particular leader or instructor; everyone in the group brings something different, everyone in the group has a different energy level, and everyone should be able to feed off of the energy level to accomplish a great workout.

A Word about Muscle-Heads, Meat-Heads, and Gym Rats

Let me put one of the old gym myths to rest right now. Not everyone who looks like a muscle- head or "gym rat" or bodybuilder is an idiot. Not everyone who grunts a little bit because they are using a heavy weight is a jerk. Matter of fact, in most cases these are very nice and extremely knowledgeable people who have experience you could learn from. Challenge your judgment and prejudice - just because someone is packing on more muscle than the "normal" person does not mean they are going to be angry or dismissive if you ask them for a spot or a question. In fact, they'll probably be flattered.

I have met male and female bodybuilders in the gym who come from all different professions. Not only were they professionals in different fields of work, but some of them possessed what I call a "PhD in Gymistry". People like this have been working out for so long that they have a vast understanding of and knowledge about the human body, dieting, and working out. To give them just a little bit more credit, it was the" gym rat" and" meat head" who were the first personal trainers. Do not be afraid to walk up to any of these people and ask them a question about anything having to do with working out or dieting because they're probably going to have a better answer for you than most certified personal trainers.

If you are person who is nervous about approaching another gym member for assistance, then ask someone you know is a personal trainer or a manager of the gym. There may be someone working behind the front desk who can give you assistance for a couple of sets, or they may be able to introduce you to a member who can, making it easier for you to connect with someone. There were many times I asked female gym members that I knew to give me some assistance. The small element of risk that my spotter was not strong enough to move the weight if I failed gave me a bit more energy to complete the task. For example, I have loaded up the bench press with 315 - 350 pounds and asked a small female member to give me a spot. During this time I've experienced a different energy – one of necessity – that allowed me to be stronger than if I had a male partner spotting me. If you are a gentleman, be respectful in the way you approach a woman in the gym, if you are going to ask her for assistance. Make her understand that you are not trying to pick her up for a date or anything unusual; the same goes for women asking men for a spot.

Another alternative to mix it up is to ask multiple people for spots on different exercises. So for one set or exercise, ask one person, and then when you get ready to do your next set ask a different person to give you assistance. Repeat this process until you've had four or five different people spotting you throughout one workout. This helps assure others that it really is about the spot, not a pick-up. And you've found potential new workout partners, or at

Success in One Day for the Rest of Your Life!

the very least, you're interacting with more people, which should make you excited about going to the gym regularly.

Make a Rut List

Getting back to creating fresh workouts: when you're stuck in a rut, find something that is new to your mind and body. Obviously, if you are doing the same thing every day, you are in a rut. If you're mixing it up but still feeling "blah" about your workouts, try keeping a record of what you're doing for a week. I don't typically recommend writing down anything that has to do with workouts, but if you can't figure out whether you're in a rut or not, it may help to write down the exercises and equipment you have used. Use this list to evaluate how you're treating your workouts and the pattern you are stuck in. You might also figure out if you're stuck in a rut by considering whether you get as sore as you used to when you started the workout. Once you figure out your rut pattern, at your next few workouts, do not touch a piece of equipment or do any exercise from your "rut list". If your "rut list" is large, and the amount of equipment you have in your gym is limited, cut your workout in half. Doing this will guarantee your workout is changed.

Or, if the rut list doesn't work for you, changing your workout can be as easy as not repeating the same stances or grips you use for each exercise: feet directly underneath shoulders for every leg exercise or hands always in the exact same position vis-à-vis

101

shoulders. To break out of the rut, change your hand position, change your foot position - and do not repeat them for every exercise. I use this idea with my clients all the time, and I call it searching for fresh muscle strands. When you're searching for fresh muscle strands, you may find your strength will decrease a bit. The decrease in muscle strength should be exciting and new to you. Also, a new lactic acid build up should occur in your muscles. This is an indication you have left your rut, at least for a day.

Another way to deal with the rut list, is to work it in sections. Maybe for your first week or two, avoid the top fourth of your "rut list" and do not touch those machines or do those exercises for two weeks. After this, do the same with another section of your rut list. Keep working through in this manner until you've completely changed the way you workout. Or, try setting the gym up into four zones, one week per zone, and then stay out of that zone for the entire week. You'll be forced to come up with creative substitutes for exercises within the zone you eliminate, but this will ensure a different workout for at least six weeks. I say six weeks because if you work through four zones of elimination, when you get back to your actual rut workout the workout will no longer be a rut. The workout is "different" again.

Use the Free Weights

Often, during an introductory gym tour, new members are shown how to use a few specific machines, and the sense of familiarity they feel causes them to want to go back to those same machines. The zone principle described above will help force you to enter and learn about other sections of the gym that you may not be comfortable or confident in - yet. The free weight section of the gym usually falls into this "other section" category, because many people, and particularly women, are nervous about using the free weights at the gym. Many gyms perpetuate the fear by putting the free weights in a small box in the back corner of the facility. That adds a physical/spatial barrier to the social barriers that may already be in place.

Whatever the setup, challenge yourself to become familiar with the free weight section because working with free weights builds a different type of muscle and strength than you can get from other equipment because you have to lift and carry the weights to a bench or open space and then back to a rack. During this process of lifting and carrying, the core and stabilizer muscles around your mid-section are working. You are getting a much fuller range of motion than the push-pull movement available on machines. This, in turn, contributes to your ability to sculpt your muscles the way you prefer, not just the way the machines are set up. When I was a bodybuilder, it was imperative to use free weights in my workouts leading up to a competition. And though not everyone is trying to become a bodybuilder, free weights can still add wonderful shape to the average person. So don't get caught in the rut of using machines as a dominant part of your workout. These machines, when used exclusively or predominantly, build Domenic strands of muscle. What this means is that in one direction, on one plane of motion, you can be really strong. But if you take the movement out of this power strand of muscle, the strength decreases exponentially. Working in the free weights section of a gym helps to prevent this from happening.

If the muscles are trained to move in linear fashion, the supporting muscles will be underdeveloped, and underdeveloped muscles or stabilizers are more likely to fail during an awkward movement. Awkward movements are those that we do every day – bending to pick up a pencil on the floor or playing tag with our children. These simple, but awkward, movements can sometimes lead to a slipped disc or other back injury if your supporting muscles are weak. Supporting muscles can be built and made stronger faster by working in a free weight area. You may have heard the saying "farm strong", and that is referring to strength that is not only able to move weight in straight push/pull lines, but also to accommodate awkward movements such as throwing from side to side or lifting and reaching positions. Every lift in the free weight area is going to be awkward; every lift will test and build on your stabilizer muscles; and every lift will engage and strengthen your core. Make your workouts fresh and exciting by visiting the free weight area of your gym.

Use the Other Equipment

What is left beyond the free weights and machines? Usually, a stretching area. And the equipment here – which can include stability balls, medicine balls, lightweight exercise bars, pull up racks, sit up racks, bosu, and sometimes even kettle bells -- lends itself to all kinds of interesting exercises. Creating a workout that only uses the equipment in the stretching area of your gym will be extremely exciting and new. The great part about using this type of equipment is that it doesn't matter how strong or how weak your muscles may be. The simple change in the workout will almost guarantee new muscle soreness. And muscle soreness equates to gains in strength, which means you are implementing successful workouts. There are literally thousands of exercise variations for the equipment listed above that exceed the scope of this book, but an internet search of any of those pieces of equipment will give you a feel for the tremendous range of options. Try some out, asking for assistance from someone in the gym if you don't quite understand the intended motion.

People sometimes think that if they don't do the same exercises that originally increased their muscle tone and strength that something will go horribly wrong. But in thinking this, we lose our freedom to be creative, to challenge our bodies and minds. There will be no harm done by not using the machines or free weights section of the gym and using the stretching area instead, or vice versa. If anything, by the time you get back to the areas you are used to at the gym, you'll end up having even more strength because of the changes you've made. Change is good! By changing we build our repertoire of exercises which will last us a lifetime. We build a spectrum of exercises that can be called upon for rainy days or sunny days, when we're ultra-fit or even injured. There's no reason to stop working out, so long as you have an open mind about your exercises.

Chapter 8: Finding a Workout Partner

I mentioned workout partners in the previous chapters, and here I'd like to go into a little more detail about the benefits of finding someone to work out with and provide some ideas about what to look for - and avoid - when selecting a partner. When it clicks, a workout partner can serve as a great motivational tool, providing inspiration and energy to get you over the rough spots when you lose focus or "just don't feel like it today". A workout partner makes you accountable to another person, and when we feel accountability or obligation, we have a tendency to follow through. Working out with someone else can also change your performance level because of the positive energy which is created in the interchange of ideas and support. And a little friendly competition never hurt either. Whether the measure is pounds or inches lost, or number of pull ups performed, having someone to work with/against is great for building positive motivation, ramping up a workout, and getting better response from your muscles.

So How Should I Choose?

There are several criteria on which you can base your selection of a workout partner. The ideal workout partner for you will:

- Be self-motivated
- Have his or her own goals set
- Already be involved in a workout routine or at a gym
- Have a similar schedule to you
- Have goals that are similar to yours
- Have a positive attitude
- Be a little bit stronger than you.

When selecting a workout partner, we try to find someone who is very motivated about working out and has established his or her own goals for health and fitness so that you don't end up having to lead someone or pull them along. If you choose a workout partner who is not excited about getting fit or who has not established their own goals, your partner will likely lose focus or commitment after a short period of time – and that can lead to lost momentum. You may be all fired up about your workout and then your workout partner just stops. And unfortunately, lack of motivation is infectious sometimes. Workout partners should share the burden of motivating each other. If you have to drag someone along it drains your energy because you're using twice the energy to motivate two people. The same reasoning is behind the idea of choosing someone who is already working out or at the gym. By finding someone already at your gym, you avoid trying to convince someone to buy a membership, or to show up every day for their workouts. You can observe other members in the gym you think you may want to work out with, or even post a request on the gym bulletin board.

When I mention having similar goals, I am concerned with making sure that, even though you are your own journeys, you are heading in the same general direction. So, for instance, try not to choose a workout partner who needs more work on their legs when you need more work on your upper body. Or that weight loss is the ultimate goal for both of you, rather than building mass. It's too hard to tailor joint workouts to divergent goals, and your partnership will likely soon fizzle. Similarly, your workout partner should be on the same basic schedule as you are for workout times. That can mean morning/evening or frequency of workouts. It is not a good idea to partner up with a person who travels a lot for work if you do not travel for work, because you will be left with a lot of solo workouts. If you both travel a lot, the partnership can still work if you hold each other accountable for the workouts. What I mean by this is that any workouts you are not able to accomplish together should still be done individually – and each partner should be held accountable for their portion of the workout schedule. This helps to keep your workouts on pace: you do not want a workout partner who is always ready to do a chest workout when it's time to do a leg workout. If this happens, you are more likely to choose to workout that is less difficult or a muscle group that is less painful to work on.

Another rule I like to use when trying to choose a workout partner is to find a partner who is 5 to 10% stronger than you are in your training. Having a workout partner who is a little stronger than you gives you a place to work toward. Obviously if everyone looked for someone stronger, one party would always be disappointed, but we balance the partnership by looking for someone stronger in some areas but weaker in others. This way you do not feel like you are always trying to keep up, nor does your partner always dominate the workouts. Moreover, it is not a good mental experience to always be the underdog in the gym: a lack of motivation will likely slowly creep into your workout. Conversely, if you are always the strongest in the workout, you will start decreasing the weight you would normally do or decreasing the amount of energy you would normally put into your own workout.

In the past I've always tried to find workout partners who were as strong as or stronger than I was in some aspect of the workout. They may be stronger on the machines or in the free weight area, in cardio or in core, but they will likely be weaker than you in at least one of these areas. Having to keep up with someone with greater strength pushes you to do more and to be better and it also gives you something to look forward to. Now of course, if your partner is 5 or 10% stronger than you, and they're doing what they're supposed to be doing in the gym, they may stay 5 or 10% stronger than you. You may stay 5 or 10% stronger than your workout partner in other aspects of the exercises. Even so, the intent is to pull each other up to a higher level of overall fitness.

And finally, if you are able to find someone with most of the other characteristics on the list, he or she will also hopefully be someone with a positive attitude – about working out and life in general. The whole rationale for having a workout partner is to provide encouragement and support in reaching your goals; you don't want to have to be a therapist, coach, cheerleader, or expend any additional energy if you are not receiving the same in kind. If your partner is an "I can't" person and repeatedly brings you down rather than buoying you up, try to find a more positive workout partner.

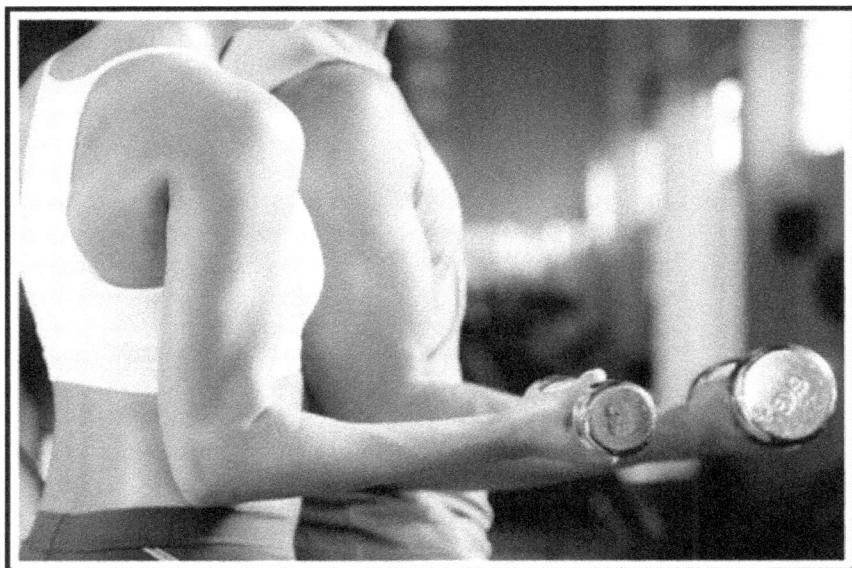

Partners as Partners?

When people think about tackling fitness goals, they often want to enlist the help and support of their spouse, significant other, or "partner". After all, this person is already very involved in your life, has your best interests at heart, and would be happy to see you fit and healthy. However, in my experience as a trainer, I have seen that having a spouse or a family member as a workout partner is not the ideal situation, for a few reasons. First, for male/female couples, the fitness goals for each member of the dyad are different. Most women want to lose weight and get smaller, while many men are looking to build muscle and strength. Eventually the workout plans must diverge to meet these different needs, and the partnership suffers.

Second, though a team mentality can be tremendously motivating, it can also hold back one or both partners. If your workout partner is a spouse and we assume that he or she is therefore someone who's feelings and choices you respect, you may be more likely to go along with a decision to skip the workout in favor of something less healthy, or to forego a workout if your partner is not around. I have spousal clients who would both cancel their workout if one of them was feeling ill. If the wife was sick, the husband would not come to the session. Or if the husband was traveling or had something going on, the wife would not come. The team mentality backfires in this situation by fostering "all or nothing" thinking about working out.

And finally, when you have a spouse or family member as a workout partner, your different roles, expectations, and energies from the various parts of your life collide. Working out with a spouse means the argument that happens at home carries over into the gym and saps energy. A miscommunication about an exercise in the gym carries over into your home life. Any carryover tension detracts from an experience which should be happy and fun. Working out for many people is their daily getaway! Obviously this is not always the case, but I've seen it enough to advise against couples workout pairings – for the benefit of your home life and your health and fitness goals. The easiest way to avoid this scenario is to find two different workout partners. That way you can still share the health and fitness experience, but bring different perspectives and energy to it.

Means of Motivation

So once you've selected a workout partner, then what? Motivate your workout partner -- and ask him or her to motivate you -- before you ever get to the gym. You can use texting, e-mails, social network sites, telephone calls, and so on to keep in contact with your workout partner. Continual contact with a workout partner means greater support - and fewer surprises that may lead to a missed workout day. Moreover, keeping in contact with your workout partner can help you with dietary motivation. Use your workout partner to discuss your latest workout, your eating for the day (good and bad), and any fitness related successes or challenges.

The more resources you can find, the less likely you'll "fall off the wagon" when temptation strikes.

Another idea is to join some sort of fitness blog. I tell my clients to "blog your fitness" on my website http://www.ImCloudFit.com. Daily engagement with your fitness promotes those conscious decisions about what you do and eat, so your journey stays on course. Fitness should be a game, and games are always more fun with others. You should not feel alone on your journey for better health and fitness even though it is a personal journey. Even if you do not have a workout partner, you can find someone else to talk to who is excited and motivated about fitness. Blogging your fitness on different fitness websites will help you to learn and educate yourself about different things fitness related. When you are more educated about fitness it becomes easier to have something to talk about with a workout partner when you have one.

Excuses, Excuses

So what is the opposite of motivation? Excuses. Because working out, getting fit, and eating healthy is hard work that requires dedicated effort and commitment, we sometimes make excuses about why we cannot succeed in reaching our goals. On some occasions when you call your workout partner to set up a workout time, they're going to make excuses about why they shouldn't or can't go. Give your workout partner the benefit of the doubt, but make sure you check them on their excuses. If the excuses are frequent then you probably want to start looking for another workout partner. Very seldom do excuse-oriented people turn into fabulous workout partners, because people who start making excuses about working out will continue to make excuses. The excuses will become more frequent until you find maybe you'll start making your own excuses for why you can't go to the gym.

Personally, I love going to the gym. On a few occasions I've had workout partners say they're not going to make it to the gym for our scheduled session. As the words were coming out of their mouths, "I will not be there today," I felt like my fire was stolen. Most times I could push myself and make myself do what needed to be done – going to the gym anyway. But there have been a few occasions where I've not gone to the gym because my workout partner bailed on a particular day. Negative workout partners steal your motivation and it can happen very quickly. This is why we are always trying to solidify the fact we can motivate ourselves. So if and when the time comes when a workout partner has other things to do, we can still accomplish our goal for the day, to keep working toward a longer-term goal.

Don't Try Too Hard

I've tried to lay out some tips to consider when choosing a workout partner, but all of that said, I believe some of the best workout partners I've ever had I discovered by accident in the gym, just by mingling with other members. It can be something you're not actively seeking, but that seems to fall into your lap because you've put yourself in a good position by being where you need to be to reach your goals. I've been at the gym and had other members come up to me to ask a question about an exercise or diet plan and without trying, I found myself with a new workout partner for a short time. The idea of asking different people for help plays a role here too. If you can find a workout partner in this manner it can be a great new motivating experience for the both of you. Remember too that a workout partner does not have to be for life. I have never worked with a workout partner for more than about two years. When you stay with a workout partner for too long, you begin to think alike and you can become stagnant in your workouts. Again, in order to stay motivated in the gym it has to be fun, fresh and exciting. If any of these elements go away because you're bored with your workout partner, it's okay to change workout partners.

Finally, put yourself first when you are thinking about choosing a workout partner. This may sound selfish, but there is no point in committing to a workout partner just to be nice or because you feel sorry for someone – your objective in having a workout partner is to push and motivate you and to keep your workouts exciting. Put yourself first when choosing a workout partner because at the end of the day it's you who has to answer for any failures or disappointments. If you can find the right match for your goals, personality, schedule, and fitness level, having a workout partner offers the potential for helping you to reach your fitness goals much faster – and more enjoyably – than if you continued alone.

Chapter 9: Hiring A Trainer

From the Start

I am a firm believer that you will achieve better results – in mind, body, and pocket – if you train yourself rather than hiring a gym-based trainer.   As I've detailed, many of these trainers are either unqualified or uninterested in your personal success.   But there are some good ones out there, and if you can't start the small changes described here by yourself, then by all means, hire a personal trainer. Because having a starting point, having a motivational partner if you cannot do it yourself, is better than nothing at all. If you do reach the conclusion that you would benefit from having a personal trainer, be sure to keep in perspective the reason you have a personal trainer (to help motivate you and hold you accountable) and what you will still need to take responsibility for (making incremental changes to your diet and activity patterns at home).   This chapter will provide you with tips on what to look for when selecting a trainer.

After You've Been Training Yourself

You may also have success with training yourself but still reach a point – the proverbial wall – where you would like help to continue on your journey to health and fitness. Guess what? Now you have money saved because you've been training yourself and you can hire a personal trainer. You may be asking yourself, "Well, why didn't I just get a personal trainer from the beginning?" The difference is that now you have education and experience; you have a different point of view. Now you have knowledge of what a personal trainer should be able to do to help you jumpstart your progress. If you have knowledge of your body, human anatomy, muscle structure, dieting and healthy eating, then you can better evaluate the level of professionalism and education of any potential personal trainers. There are too many personal trainers in the health and fitness industry who look really good and who passed a certification of some kind, but who also do not have as much knowledge and experience as they should. Moreover, there are many personal trainers out there who are not worth the money that you are paying them -- or the gym to which you belong. But now that you have the knowledge and experience gained from training yourself, you can recognize a sub-par personal trainer – and avoid him or her!

I believe the aphorism that knowledge is power, but not the adage that ignorance is bliss. You should know something about your personal trainer before engaging him. At least if you have been your own personal trainer for 40 or 50 or 60 sessions, and you've paid yourself for the education of being your own personal trainer, you will be able to go through a workout or an assessment with a prospective personal trainer and immediately identify the value and expertise of that personal trainer. I've had people come to me who believed the personal trainer they had before me was knowledgeable because s/he was nice. There is a difference between knowledgeable and nice. Would you let a "nice" doctor perform surgery? It's an extreme example, but the point is the same: a personal trainer who is nice but has little knowledge or experience is putting you at risk for injury. At this point you have enough education to make an informed decision – which may mean telling a given personal trainer (and perhaps the fitness facility) to take a walk.

Choosing Wisely

A good trainer can be a tremendous asset, worth every dollar for the motivation, experience, knowledge, and attitude they bring to the training sessions. A bad trainer, on the other hand, can be a waste of money or downright dangerous, putting you at risk for injury. So how do you choose? In the next few sections I'll give you some tips on what to look for and avoid, using examples from my years of watching and interacting with other trainers. In all cases, you should avoid walking into a gym or fitness facility and asking for a personal trainer. The personal trainer they select will be assigned because he or she happens to be there at the facility – not because he or she is the most knowledgeable personal trainer or the one who best fits your needs; they just want to set you up with a personal trainer because you are paying them $35 per session.

Knowledge and Experience

As I've mentioned, working with a trainer who is not properly educated or experienced can put you at risk for injury, which is why an evaluation of their knowledge and practice is much more important than any certification they may have. For instance, at one point I worked at a relatively new facility that hired a trainer who had gotten his certification about a year prior. We'll call him Fred. Fred carried himself with the confidence (bordering arrogance) of someone who had been in the business for decades. Over the weeks, it became obvious that this trainer was watching me with my clients to learn from me. We all learn from others, and I have no problem with that, but we also have to know when and how to correctly apply what we learn. Fred was learning from me, and I even put him through several workouts to make sure he could understand and apply my exercises to his clientele properly. However, Fred's ego was more developed than his learning, and soon he was boasting that he was a better trainer than I was. I don't waste my time or energy on that kind of nonsense, but I *was* incensed by how Fred was using what he had learned from me, which showed total lack of understanding of the who, when, and how of certain exercises.

Here's the thing: Any exercise I introduce to a client has been tried and tested for months if it's something no one else has done before. Fred was selling exercises he was using with particular clients as things he had complete knowledge of and personal experience with. He had no regard for or awareness of clients' differing needs and abilities. Fred was having female clients doing overhead presses and dead lifts – power lifting moves -- without even understanding these exercises himself. With the confidence he exuded, Fred "sold" these moves to clients, but he did not have enough education to understand that the information he was giving them was too advanced, or in some cases, just plain wrong. He used the exact same workout for every single client, male or female. I complained to the manager/operators of this particular fitness facility, but they did nothing about the dangerous situation. They weren't concerned about the client; they were only concerned about the client paying money. Five of Fred's clients ended up with severe injuries, and three of them ended up working out with me. We had to rehabilitate injured muscles and muscle imbalances before we could move on, which is not what these clients had intended to pay a trainer for help with.

I provide this example to illustrate the importance of using your own knowledge and experience to assess the competence of a trainer – and to challenge the trainer to back up his confidence with experience. Be aware of being used as a guinea pig by your personal trainer. The trainer should know what she or he is doing – and have had experience training a variety of people at different levels – before you become her or his client. Investing the time to interview and have a trial session with prospective personal trainers will save you a great deal down the road. Before I took on Fred's clients, I interviewed them to see if they were a good fit for me as well. When

I took them on as clients, I asked them to do their best to forget everything they learned from Fred, so that they could be open to my way of training and could begin to understand what a truly knowledgeable, understanding, caring, personable, professional, personal trainer is really like.

The Used Car Salesman

Like Fred, many personal trainers have more confidence or pride than is warranted by their skill or experience (the truly experienced trainers are usually pretty humble). And many of them are smooth talkers. Don't forget that gym-based trainers receive incentives from the gyms that are based on quantity, not quality. And so you get trainers with a used car salesman mentality and style. They're interested in being the top salesman, the trainer who sells the most sessions, month after month. And following through on those sales in the form of training sessions is secondary.

There was another incident at the same particular facility that illustrates this nicely. One night I was standing behind the front desk of the gym when a woman came in who was very upset. I had no idea what she was so upset about, but one of the other employees behind the desk went to get one of the managers. Apparently her trainer, let's call him Jim said she "would not succeed without him" in her weight loss and fitness goals. I don't believe in all of my years of being a personal trainer or being around a gym I have ever heard a personal trainer tell a client something so rude and manipulative. But it fits perfectly with the used car salesman mentality, where the trainer is out to make a sale.

When the gym operator reached the desk and asked her what the problem was, she immediately demanded her money back for the training session and cancelled her gym membership. The operator's husband went over to Jim and suggested he apologize to this client, but I suspect this was for the sake of the fitness center, since there were many members in the facility this night and people were becoming aware of the situation. But the woman, to her credit, wouldn't even hear it. This type of conduct is absolutely unforgivable, and had it been my facility, Jim would have been fired immediately. But then again, a personal trainer with that type of attitude would never make it at the I'm Core Fit studios in the first place. Jim was eventually fired when he turned his big mouth on the owners and cursed out the manager's wife and the operator himself, but had he continued to abuse only his clients, this unprofessional personal trainer would probably still be working at the same facility today.

So here's the point: The sales ability of a personal trainer has nothing to do with his or her competence as a personal trainer. Make sure the gym and/or personal trainer you enter into a contract with are concerned with quality more than quantity. Don't let a personal trainer smooth talk you into thinking he or she is the best, or that you need him to reach your goals. The rest of this book should have proven to you that you don't.

Pushing Through the Pain

Another telltale sign of a poor personal trainer is one who uses the words "push through it" too often. If you are working with a personal trainer who insists you "push through" every ache and pain, you are probably going to end up with a long-term injury. There are some pains you should not push through, even if they seem to be small at the time. There is a difference between muscle stress pain and pain that can cause a back injury, muscle tear, joint stress, or so on. The important thing to remember is that the small nagging pain you may be having while you are exercising will probably not manifest itself completely while you are "pushing through". It's when you least expect it, after you go home and are getting out of your car or are bending down to pick up a dropped pencil and your back "goes out". Small nagging pains can be a sign of improper form or overuse, and should be investigated or accommodated, rather than ignored.

I've had clients come into my studio or the gym with a slight nagging pain and I've either completely modified their workout or sent them home. Or in other cases, if they are not completely over having an illness, I'll send them home. I do this because it is not worth being unable to work out for a month or two because you happen to "push through" at the wrong time. It is better and safer all the way around to just go home for a day or two and give your body some rest. Then get back to the workout and hit it hard when you've recovered. A lot of personal trainers feel they are losing money if they send the client home, but this is short-sighted. Losing one day to a nagging pain is better than losing the six or eight weeks it would take to heal an injury. And a good personal trainer should be able to change a workout on the fly to accommodate any pain.

On rainy days I am particularly sensitive to clients' little annoying pains, creaks, and pops, as these may be signs that the weather has caused muscles or joints to stiffen. If a client comes in on a rainy day with an unusual complaint about a particular muscle group or joint, I'll have her warm up and stretch to see if it works itself out. If it doesn't, and I choose not to send the client home, then the workout changes to a different group of muscles. Usually just by changing the focus of the muscle group or the particular exercise, clients find that the annoying little pain has gone away. So there is really no need to "push through" during a workout if your trainer has the ability to be responsive and creative.

Cell Phone Use

There is a disturbing trend among the younger generation of personal trainers to carry and use a mobile phone while training clients. In my eyes, this is unforgivably disrespectful to a client.

There is no reason for a personal trainer to even have a phone on them during your training session, let alone use it to text someone or access the internet. Simple common sense tells us that if a trainer is texting while training, he or she is not paying attention to the client – who could pull a muscle, get a back injury, drop a weight, or have any other kind of accident before a phone-holding personal trainer could react. If your personal trainer is texting or talking on the phone during your training session, fire him or her right away. I am completely astounded that personal trainers do not have enough good sense and respect to focus on their clients for a mere 30 minutes without using their phones. If this is your personal trainer, why waste your money? Why waste your time? It doesn't matter whether you are paying $5 or $105 per session. It is still your money, paid for a service that should be professional.

Correcting Muscle Imbalances

Personal trainers should be paying attention to clients for many reasons. In addition to insuring proper form, motivating us to give maximum effort, and preventing injury, a good trainer's well-honed eye will help to identify muscle imbalances. We all have these, and if a personal trainer is not watching for them, these imbalances become amplified. Think of it like a small tree growing near a fence. If while this small sapling is growing it comes in contact with the fence, it has to change direction slightly in order to keep growing. It doesn't mean the tree will not take root or continue to grow, it just means the tree grows on a different path. Similarly, the muscle imbalances you do not correct early by moving the tree or the fence, so to speak, will continue to follow this "crooked" trajectory.

As a client you need to recognize whether your personal trainer is looking for and correcting your muscle imbalances. Again, we all have muscle imbalances so this should be happening with 100% of a trainer's clients. Most of our muscle imbalances show through our feet and then work their way up. Therefore, a muscle imbalance located in your back may manifest itself in the way your heels raise or whether you duck walk, which may in turn manifest itself as one knee or the other pulling in or pushing out during a squat.

TRAINERS TIP: If you are training yourself, you need to be looking out for the same muscle imbalances. These muscle imbalances are not easy to correct and for the most part are only corrected over long periods of time. Here is an example: if you are getting ready to do a squat, square your feet up to your shoulders so your foot/shoulder alignment is perfect. Your arms are straight down on your thighs. As you squat, your hands come up to eye level. If when you do this squatting motion your heels come up off the floor, you have muscle imbalances. If during the squat one or both of your knees push in or out, or you can't keep your upper body from pushing forward, these are signs of muscle imbalances. In order to correct these muscle imbalances, your focus should be on readjusting your feet constantly and squatting as if you are sitting in a chair.

There are a few more subtle muscle imbalances that are a little bit harder to see. One is what I call the hip shift. The "hip shift" is when your hips make a small movement left or right on the way up or down during a squat. Your hips should be completely locked in place traveling in a straight up-and-down motion. Another sign of imbalance is the "ducking" of the feet, when your feet push out in duck-like fashion while you are squatting. This is usually attributable to tight hamstrings and calves, which can sometimes also cause the feet to roll over from the outside in. If you are acting as your own personal trainer you should be looking for these muscle imbalances. Moreover, a personal trainer should be able to recognize these muscle imbalances every single time.

A good professional personal trainer should be able to recognize these muscle imbalances and constantly be reminding the client of proper form. This is why a personal trainer must pay attention to your every move and every exercise, especially if you are new to working out. If he or she does not pay attention to your every move, they will miss the opportunity to learn about your body's performance. Trainers have an advantage over you in identifying your muscle imbalances because to you these motions feel normal. When a personal trainer notices and corrects muscle imbalances, you should feel awkward performing the same movement in the corrected position.

Watch for Workout Routines or Ruts

When you are working with a personal trainer and you feel you are stuck in a rut, don't be afraid to request different workouts. The trainer should not be offended because you've realized you are stuck in a rut. If she is, then she may not have the knowledge to get out of the rut herself. As when you're training yourself, at all cost stay out of the rut – even if it means finding a new trainer or training yourself for a while. Asking your personal trainer to give you a different workout is going to test her knowledge and ability to be a great personal trainer. She should rise to the occasion and be excited she is challenged to do something new.

Really good personal trainers rarely get requests from clients to mix up the workout plan because these trainers keep their clients guessing about what workout they're going to do for any particular day. I really mess with my clients if they think they can recognize a pattern forming in the way I train them. If they come into my studio and suggest we are going to work a particular body part, I will start with that body part and then completely change the workout on them. This tactic keeps clients and their muscles guessing every time.

My philosophy is that clients should never be aware of a workout pattern or progression that would allow their mind and body to prepare ahead of time for the workout. From my experience, if a client knows the workout ahead of time, the performance level during the workout is decreased. The muscles prepare themselves for the work to be done and seek the path of least resistance. Moreover, there's a bit of motivation lost if you know nothing is going to be fresh and new during a given workout. If you woke up every morning and knew you were going to have a banana and a bowl of cereal for breakfast, I guarantee your excitement about this pairing would diminish over time.

Trainer/Client Relationship

A few my clients call me Coach. I believe the words *coach* and *personal trainer* mean two different things. Yes, I am a personal trainer, but my philosophy is to coach my clients through every movement they perform in order to educate them mind, body, and soul. I am constantly coaching my clients through their exercise movements and readjusting when they fall back into bad habits. We could use a little kid who's just learning T-ball for an example. As the small child is developing, there has to be constant reinforcement in the movements they're making until those movements become natural to the child. When dealing with muscle imbalances the same principles apply. I coach the client, reinforce and re-correct the movements in every exercise until it becomes a natural fluid movement.

In addition to being a coach, I believe your personal trainer should be a friend, in terms of being supportive, ethical, caring, and educating. If your personal trainer is not performing all of these roles to your satisfaction, then you should find one who will. I know sometimes clients do not want to be bothered about the gym once they leave, but for me, after-hours follow up is a sign of a good trainer. By follow up I mean contacting clients not just for workout scheduling, but to see how they may be doing periodically, or after a particularly intense workout. If your personal trainer is only concerned with you as a client from the time you walk into the gym to the time your session is over, you may want to reevaluate the relationship. I'm not saying the personal trainer who does not contact you periodically is a bad trainer. Only that I believe a personal trainer who shows a little initiative in how they care about their clients is better. A better personal trainer is one who shows you it is not all about getting your money. An excellent personal trainer lets you know he or she appreciates the opportunity to be able to help you reach your fitness goals. An excellent personal trainer will have contact with you as a client once or twice a month without it being a scheduled workout day. This contact could be an e-mail, phone call, a visit or it could be just walking up to you to say hi when you're in the gym working out by yourself.

If you have a personal trainer you consider a friend, but you are carrying the friendship, your personal trainer is not for you. By carrying the friendship, I mean that you are the one asking (or at least hearing) about everything in the trainer's life, without reciprocation. For example, I've worked in fitness facilities from morning to night and heard personal trainers who, for the entire workout of every client, repeat the same story over and over again. Not only are they recounting what they did over the weekend – what they drank, who they partied with – during the process they are completely ignoring their clients. I've seen some of their clients give hints they would like to talk about their weekend, but they can't get a word in edgewise. Personal trainers get paid to listen to clients. Listening is how we understand the mindset of our clients so we can better serve them and help them reach their goals. This is impossible if the trainer's mouth is moving the whole time. A personal trainer's weekend exploits are irrelevant to a paying client. Usually the "talkers" are easy to spot, so it's a good idea to observe potential personal trainers before signing a contract. Check out how they interact with their clients, or ask their clients what they think about the personal trainer.

Another way to evaluate the quality of a client/trainer relationship is to think about how you feel before a workout. If you feel anxiety about the workout when you think about visiting your personal trainer, he or she is not for you. As a client you should be happy and motivated to go to every session, and at the very least you should feel obligated and accountable because your personal trainer is making him or herself available to you. The relationship should be both friendly and professional. I have clients today who say they consider me a part of their family, but when they come into my studio and it's time to work, we all know that I am the boss. When clients come into my studio, they understand they are there for a particular reason and that is to increase their health and fitness. Though I am amazingly honored when someone says I am like a part of their family, I also keep in perspective my duties, knowing that my role in that family is to make sure the client is getting a great professional health and fitness service.

How Long Do I Work with a Personal Trainer?

Of course the answer to this varies with each person's aptitude for learning how to exercise and motivate themselves, in direct connection with the type of relationship established between client and trainer. There's a certain amount of education your personal trainer should be giving to you as a client each and every time you have a workout session, so you are able to perform your workouts on your own. A good personal trainer educates clients about all facets of health and fitness. There should be constant information coming from a personal trainer about motivation strategies, creativity in exercises, dietary hints, coaching, and so on. A good professional personal trainer should be preparing the client for independence during each workout session. If you have a personal trainer who is not giving you this type of knowledge, then he or she may be stringing you on for a paycheck. Don't become dependent on using a personal trainer to help you reach your health and fitness goals; depend on your trainer to fill in the gaps of your knowledge and experience so you can be a better independent trainer of yourself.

I have nothing against a personal trainer who is able to retain clients for one, two, or three years or more. But there is a problem with a personal trainer who has a client who cannot perform on their own after about a year. This is one of my basic rules in personal training. Clients should be able to continue their workouts, self-motivation, and progress towards their personal goals after one year with a personal trainer. If after a successful year you choose to stay with the trainer because you've built a friendship and relationship, wonderful. I've had clients stay with me for over three years, because of a relationship and friendship we have built, but they are able to continue reaching their fitness goals without use of my services. I've also had clients work out with me for less than a year because of financial reasons. I've had clients who come and work out for 20 or 30 sessions, stop using my services for while, and then come back for refreshers. There is no "right" answer for how long you should use a personal trainer, just make sure the services and education you are receiving are right.

Having read this book, I hope you now believe that you can succeed without a personal trainer. As an educated consumer in the field of health and fitness, you should be able to make good decisions about whether to start or continue using personal training services without fear of being lost. You should have enough knowledge to continue coaching and motivating yourself to continually set and reach new fitness goals.

Chapter 10: Testimonials

Throughout this book I have thrown out a lot of information based on my extensive experience as a fitness consultant. I include the following stories from some of my clients to illustrate the power of a good fitness consultant, and to inspire you to be or find that trainer for yourself, to improve your health, your fitness, and your life.

Michelle's Story

The year was 2005 and I had never truly committed to exercise. Before I had a family I didn't feel the need to exercise, but by this time I'd already had two children and I was not happy with the way I looked. I was also jealous of all the other mothers who felt comfortable going to the gym. So I decided to join my first gym. But the only way I would feel comfortable in a gym, using any equipment other than the treadmill, would be with a trainer.

The first trainer I was assigned seemed good. He came across as knowledgeable, but he wasn't always 100% committed to my session. He'd take phone calls during my session. He cancelled a lot. Eventually he was fired. By the time I was assigned a second trainer I was pregnant with my third child. He also seemed pretty knowledgeable, but he certainly didn't practice what he preached, especially when it came to nutrition.

After my third child was 7 months old I joined a new gym and was assigned Michaelson as my personal trainer. From the beginning it was obvious that Michaelson definitely knew what he was talking about. He wasn't into the cookie-cutter type of exercises that I'd seen a lot of other personal trainers doing with their clients. I trusted Michaelson's instruction and guidance much more than I did my previous trainers. Michaelson was also very well versed in the nutritional aspects of health and fitness, in conjunction with exercise.

After he branched out on his own, I followed Michaelson to his own fitness studio.

I did have a set back over a year ago, when I had surgery to reconstruct a torn ACL. I used the rehab time as an excuse to not exercise and watch my nutrition as well as I should have. I was horrified to discover I weighed the most I'd ever been, not being pregnant. Michaelson gave me the tools and encouragement to lose the weight and come back from my injury even stronger and fitter than before. I ended up losing almost 20 pounds and have never felt better about myself.

Even though I have now been with him for over four and a half years, Michaelson still encourages me to push myself. Michaelson has made me feel strong and proud to be able to do things I never thought I could. He has turned me into a competitive person in the gym. Michaelson has always challenged me to reach beyond what I think I can do. I'm always looking to get to the top of his leader-board. Prior to Michaelson going to the gym was a chore, but now I look forward to my workouts. Because of Michaelson, health and fitness has become an integral part of my lifestyle.

Michelle Speakmaster

Marc's Story

I worked out pretty regularly in college. But I was not very educated when it came to exercise. I pretty much followed my "bigger" college roommate around the gym and worked out like he did. Still, as a 6'1" guy weighing 150 lbs I did see some gains. I didn't appreciate at the time though that I was lacking a fundamental understanding of exercise, muscles/movements, and nutrition.

Flash forward 15 years (which had been pretty exercise-free) and my doctor informed me that my good cholesterol numbers are too low. By now I weighted about 165 lbs. My doctor went on to explain that aerobic exercise would help. So I began jogging. Soon enough I was bored simply jogging so I went into the gym. I immediately found myself falling back into the same routines I remembered in college and didn't feel like I was making good use of my time (or money!). My wife was already working out with Michaelson but I signed up with another trainer. I was immediately unimpressed and asked the owners if I could switch to Michaelson.

It wasn't long after that when Michaelson left and opened I'm Core Fit. I've now been training with Michaelson for about two years and it was the best decision of my life. It changed my life. In fact, I'm very proud to say that I'm an original client of Michaelson's at I'm Core Fit. Every workout with Michaelson is a challenge and I'm continually amazed that after two years he's still creating entirely new workouts that test me body and mind. I now weigh about 180 lbs and the extra weight is all muscle. Michaelson's total body approach to exercise has increased my "core" strength tremendously. I no longer suffer any lower back pain. I also have an appreciation for what I eat and when I eat. When I go into a traditional gym on my own I don't even want to work out on the machines, knowing how much I can push myself with simply an exercise ball and my own body as resistance, for example.

The simple truth is that I don't know what I'd do if I couldn't work out with Michaelson. Nobody pushes me like him and the I'm Core Fit model is fantastic. The gains for me have been as much mental as they are physical. I can't recall how many times Michaelson has pushed me forward by saying "It's all in your head Marc". My confidence has grown tremendously. I hold myself better, head high, shoulders back and that has helped me take on new challenges (e.g. work) outside of the gym.

I'd really like to find out just how many pushups and squats I've performed since joining I'm Core Fit. Probably a scary high number!

Marc Farber

Bob's Story

At 55 years old, knowing that my dad passed away at the age of 54, I made a determination that I was going to get myself into shape and lose some weight. Those were my exact goals! Having grown up tall and thin, I never dreamed I would ever have to try to lose weight, let alone be considered "obese" by the standard "height & weight" charts! Unfortunately, over the last 15 years or so I put on 35 to 40 extra pounds...mostly in my stomach area. With a very busy personal/business schedule including 50% out of town travel, I knew I needed some help to get started, but had no idea where or to whom to go. I knew I would not get what I needed by going to the local gym and running on the treadmill or other cardio machines.

I first heard about Michaelson Williams from my wife, who managed a Little Caesars pizza restaurant located next to the fitness center where Michaelson worked a few years earlier. So I went to visit Michaelson at *I'm Core Fit* for an introductory work out. After that I was ready to get started and serious about getting back in shape. That first day I could barely do a single push-up! I signed up for½ hour sessions 3 days a week ...and boy were some of those early sessions BRUTAL! It took every bit of effort I could muster up to push through...but I was determined! I would never have continued on had I not had a financial commitment (paid in advance) and been so determined to succeed with my goals. Fortunately, I stuck it out and with Michaelson's constant encouragement, insistence and 'hard love' he pushed me through the initial stage and kept me coming back each time for another "whoop'n". As I progressed, I could steadily feel myself getting stronger. My first unanticipated accomplishment was the fact that I started getting up earlier in the morning ready to go...because I was getting a better night's sleep!

Next Michaelson started his 'boot camps' three days a week, which meant that I was now working out 6 days a week (when I was in town). A main emphasis of the camp was on losing weight by eating properly in combination with the workouts. So I started an entirely new lifestyle in eating. It was at this stage that I started shedding pounds. Over the course of about 12 weeks I lost 30 pounds...while at the same time gaining muscle mass. It has been over 5 months and I have maintained my new weight and have no plans on going back where I was!

Michaelson has the type of personality that keeps you engaged and causes you to push yourself harder to reach beyond your known or planned limits. Michaelson gave me a compliment the other day that really meant a lot to me. He asked me how old I was... "Are you 51?" I responded with the correct age of 55. He proceeded to inform me that I was holding my own against some of his clients that were 10, 15 some 20 years younger! That meant a lot to me! Thanks to my determination and Michaelson's training and encouragement my body feels better and stronger than I can ever remember it feeling!

Regards, Bob Hoover

Jason's Story

I have had the distinct pleasure of incorporating the I'm Core Fit training methods into my life over the previous 3 years, and my life has changed for the better as a result. I don't look at my sessions with Michaelson as just "workouts" but as a progression and a change in lifestyle that will enable a stronger physical body and more confident mind. Learning how to treat my body has been an epiphany and I couldn't be happier with the results. And it is not just the exercise portion. It is learning how to eat, and what not to eat and drink. Many times in our sessions the conversations have turned to healthy eating habits and without the eating changes I would never have had the results I wanted. You cannot truly get healthy and strong without both the exercise and proper diet. I would say it is just as or more important to learn how to eat correctly. And how to supplement your diet.

The physical parts of our workouts have concentrated on the core. I was 39 years old when I met Michaelson and had a back issue that was running my life. Now I am 41, have a strong core band, and back problems are a thing of the past. I attribute this change to the methods I've learned from Michaelson and the I'm Core Fit way of training. Getting and keeping the body in shape starts from the core; the legs and the upper body should follow. Without a strong core there is no reason to sit there and do the usual bench press and curls that you see so many people do in the gym, without getting the results they want. That was me. I learned to lose weight but I did not know how to truly get strong and healthy. It is two

years later and I am the strongest and healthiest I've been since my college days. Every workout is focused, intense, and has purpose. And the things I learn can be brought forward for the rest of my life.

Mentally the workouts have been awakening as well. Being pushed to do things that you didn't think were possible builds confidence. I have built on each little success and continue to reach milestones. The mental aspect is a large part of that. Try "sitting against the wall" with legs at 90 degrees for over 4 minutes. The brain goes to places you didn't plan on. But learning to stay focused and in the moment can help the pain subside. And then when you get to that "time" that you hadn't reached before the confidence raises a tick. Then next time it gets a little easier. That is one thing I've come to learn. In fitness you need to be patient and realize that with consistent work and better eating habits you will get the results you want. But it takes time. You cannot expect immediate results. I think this is why so many people fail to lose weight and keep it off. The process must be trusted and time must be given to allow the results to come.

I will take what I've learned and apply it for the rest of my life. Good training habits must be learned and it helps to learn from a pro. Someone who can assist with the right methods for YOU. Everyone is different and has different needs and speeds. A good trainer realizes that and will work at the pace that is right for you. And the best thing of all is the confidence and life improvements that I have seen outside of the training sessions.

A strong core has led to a golf game I never had. A sore back used to be the norm after golf rounds. Not anymore! And my game has improved as a result of a healthy core, stronger legs, and focused mind. I also enjoy running and since my legs are stronger than ever, running now comes easier as well. I can jump higher when playing beach volleyball. I have quickness and strength that did not exist a few years ago. Even though I am older, I look and feel younger than I did 5years ago. Life is good!

Jason Paul Grieco

Janine's Story

At 43 years old, I found myself desperate, ready to give up all hope of ever losing the weight I had gained. I had reached 198 pounds and yo-yoed up and down from this weight for 10 years. Having an underactive thyroid didn't help. Thinking I could just hit the gym using the information I read from the internet and my past experience of dance and working out, I joined the gym. I was there 6 days a week and working out 1 ½ to 2 hours a day. One hour of cardio and one hour of weight lifting. I did this for 1 month and lost a whopping 1lb. Desperate, I went to the manager of the gym and told him my struggle. He suggested I meet with a trainer.

My first experience working with a trainer was great, or so I thought. He pushed me to the point that I wanted to cry. I would go home and not be able to move for over an hour in fear of passing out or getting sick. In about 3 weeks I had lost 5lbs. I am by nature a strong person, so my trainer focused in on this. He used the philosophy of using only the large muscle group which in turn would cause me to burn more fat and get faster results!

So every time we worked out we pushed the weight up more and more. And about this time in our work outs I started to notice something with his training that bothered me. He was always looking around the gym, looking for his next client or someone to talk to. I would have to ask him if I was doing the lifts correctly. He was late starting my work-outs and ended 5 minutes early. I started to feel like "just a client." Just a payment.

My last work out with him, we jumped right into dead lifts. I did 150 pound dead lifts 10 times, then jumped down and did 10 pushups. Ten more dead lifts and I felt a strange pull in my tail bone. He said it was nothing, not to worry about it; back to the pushups. When I got up to finish the dead lifts I couldn't bend my knees, my legs turned to jelly. After having me do some stretches and try a different weight lifting exercise that I could not accomplish, he sent me home. I never heard from him again. Not even a phone call or e-mail to see how I was. I was laid up for over 3 months, having injured the #5 and #6 discs in my spine.

After doing some light therapy with a chiropractor and gaining back the whole 10 pounds I had finally lost, I wanted to get back in the gym. While leaving the gym I noticed the *I'm Core Fit Studio* sign across the parking lot *10 workouts for $10 each.* I thought "What a great deal!" and went home and made the phone call. My first workout with Michaelson, I immediately noticed a difference in the training. Michaelson noticed even the small things like the position of my feet and the way I ran on my toes. The entire time I worked out Michaelson would walk around me and look at my form, correcting me as we worked. Not once did he look at the clock or look at the door as if he couldn't wait for the session to be over.

Slowly, he helped my back to heal by strengthening my core. The few times I felt pain or a pull he immediately stopped me and either corrected something I was doing wrong or said we were done for the day; my body was giving signs of stress. After, Michaelson would call or e-mail to see how I was feeling, giving me some stretches to do while at home.

With my struggle of having underactive thyroid, Michaelson has helped me overcome major pitfalls in weight loss and my metabolism, having done research for me and encouraging me to do some as well. We have found different things that have helped my metabolism kick in and help me lose weight. When we would hit a wall in my weight loss, he found something else to help. Not once did he give up on me, but instead encouraged me to change my negative thinking to positive. He has helped and continues to help me from being so hard on myself and just be proud of what I have accomplished.

One and a half years later I have lost 35lbs, my back is stronger, and I feel better and more fit. Through this time Michaelson has never treated me as a "client." Instead, he has become a friend, stepping into the trenches with me while keeping a very professional atmosphere. I believe Michaelson is a very rare trainer in the fact that he truly cares more about the person rather than the "client" (pay check).

Janine Amato

Steve's Story

Nothing but the BEST. That has been my lifelong motto. I have been training in the martial arts for 30 years and own a karate school in Raleigh named Best Karate. I train to be the best competitor, instructor, and official; I train my karate students to be the best that they can be.

When I started getting chronic injuries in karate years ago, I added weight-training to strengthen my muscles and joints. From there, I worked from 1998-2004 as a certified personal trainer and hired, supervised, and evaluated hundreds of other personal trainers for more than 40 gyms. So I know a little about people and trainers.

I met Michaelson in a gym in Raleigh in 2007. As a fellow martial artist with similar upbringings in Pennsylvania, we established an instant friendship. As I watched him with his clients and picked his brain about weight-training techniques and nutrition, I realized why he was the best in the gym. He has vast knowledge about the human body and he genuinely cares about the success of his clients.

In 2008, Michaelson wanted to leave the gym to start I'm Core Fit in a smaller setting. I invited him to use Best Karate's space because his integrity, high standards of excellence, and knowledge matched my school's philosophy. I'm Core Fit clients came in the morning and Best Karate students came in the afternoon. I observed his group classes, he observed mine. He had fiercely loyal clients who made wellness a priority in their busy lives. In 2009, I asked Michaelson to design a conditioning program for 45 members of the competitive karate team ages 5 to 55. Michaelson introduced core training for the group and made each drill fun and competitive. Despite the rigorous challenge, core training quickly became everyone's favorite hour of the week.

When I got in a rut in my own training last year, I asked Michaelson to train me to reach a new level of fitness. I went to Michaelson as a client, not as his landlord. Michaelson is creative, attentive to details, and safety-minded. He holds everyone accountable for every move done correctly and completely. He designed several food plans for me. I notice the difference in my body composition in a month. Over six months of sustained training (something that Michaelson is adamant about), I lost 5% body fat. I still train with him regularly and he continues to challenge me. Nothing but the BEST.

If this book is anything like the way Michaelson trains his clients, you are in for an eye-opening experience.

Stephen Robinson, age 45

6th degree black belt and Chief Karate Instructor

Member, AAU-USA Karate Referee Council,

Member, World Karate Confederation Referee Council

Jason Dickens Story

Throughout my adult life I considered myself to be physically fit. I worked out regularly (4-5 days a week) in a gym (weights and cardio), ran several times a week, and was an avid hiker. I had also spent 13 years in the Marines Corps where I annually performed at a first class fitness level and successfully completed various military training evolutions. Even though I was disciplined and successful, I understood my current path did not lead me to lifelong wellness. First I had yet to heal completely from a recent ACL knee reconstructive surgery, even though I had been medically released. My stamina, dexterity (balance), and flexibility were all suboptimal. And my workout recovery period and injury rehabilitations were frustrating slow. By classic western medicine standards (BMI, heart rate, blood pressure etc.) however I was deemed in great health. Moreover, most professionals deemed my "minor" concerns as middle age issues. I knew better!!

My goals were to return my reconstructed knee to pre-surgery mobility, reach and maintain a fitness level equivalent of an athlete half my age, and develop a deeper understanding of holistic wellness (body, mind, and spirit). To achieve these goals my fitness approach had to change and change drastically. This is when Michaelson William entered into my life. Michaelson's fitness philosophy simultaneously addressed all of my goals and most importantly cultivated my mental edge. Significant improvement in physical agility, balance and stamina are the hallmarks of the benefits I've realized.

Executing a perfect lower plank for over 12 minutes during I'm Core Fit "plank challenge" is one measure of how far I've advanced. Michaelson's disciplined and dynamic training philosophy which emphasizes core fitness, small and large muscle control and mental development has been a life changing experience that has impacted all aspects of my life. I have a much deeper understanding of my personal biomechanics. I've developed a capacity to design my own comprehensive training regime including integration of regular rehabilitation and injury rehabilitation. And most importantly I've learned to appreciate that fitness is truly 95% mental and 5% physical. Thank you Michaelson for your guidance and instruction over the last few years! Until the next Everest....

Jason E. Dickens

ABOUT THE AUTHOR

Michaelson William, an entrepreneur, author, and critical thinker, applies a unique philosophy and psychology when thinking about health and fitness success. Being the CEO of multiple companies, involved in martial arts since the age of 4 ½ years old, a health and fitness consultant, and an avid student of years of psychology study, he developed a unique technique called "Line of Sight" fitness training. He hopes his new ICFTS—I'm Core Fit Training System techniques will assist others to be successful in their own health and fitness.

Michaelson possesses various degrees and professional certificates from business, martial arts, personal training, and security contracting. This gives Michaelson a broad perspective on how people and the human mind react to pressure when dealing with success and failure. Michaelson continues to educate himself in the ways of human thinking and behaviors in order to help others on a successful journey in life. Michaelson has already written several books in different genres but all are based on the functionality and psychology of the human mind.

TO CONTACT THE AUTHOR, PLEASE WRITE OR EMAIL:

Michaelson Williams

306 Berlin Way

Morrisville, NC 27560

USA

(919) 673-0941

Michaelson.williams@hwfnet.com

HWFnet, LLC.

(919) 651-8006

1-855-590-8693

http://hwfnet.com

http://imcloudfit.com

OTHER MATERIAL BY MICHAELSON WILLIAMS

Books

Trainwashing: The Secrets of Positive Brain Washing

The Adventures of CT: The Children's Books for Adults

Series

Volume 1: The Beginning

Volume 2: Words of Honor

Volume 3: I Will

Volume 4: The Green Machine

Articles

Expert Author

Ezine Articles

http://ezinearticles.com/?expert=Michaelson_Williams

Blog

Blogoyle on Blogspot

http://blogoyle.blogspot.com/